Relax and Enjoy Your Baby

This, and everything else, for Jack —L.S.

For my mother, Margaret Mackay Cheney,
and my brothers, Robert and Thomas Mackay —K.M.

Contents

Introduction

I LOVE BEING a pediatrician. As my partner's daughter Katie once said, it's "funner" than I thought it would be. Watching children grow and working closely with their parents are kicks for me. When I was a resident, I saw a child in the emergency room who had a history of severe allergies—chocolate, nuts, strawberries, you name it. Her mother was a nuts and berries lady who lived in a rustic canyon near Los Angeles and ate only what she had grown or gathered herself. She firmly believed that anything natural couldn't possibly hurt you. She made a "natural" skin cream out of strawberries and rubbed it on her daughter, who, of course, broke out in hives and swelled up immediately. I knew that the reaction would clear quickly with a shot of adrenaline. I also knew that the little girl was deathly afraid of shots.

"You're going to have a shot," I said. The child drew back in terror, and I quickly added, "But I'll do my 'rash-go-away dance,' and you'll be fine in a few minutes." As the nurse administered her shot, I took out my reflex hammer and danced around, doing my imitation Indian rain dance and chanting mystical sounding noises. Not only did the little girl's reaction subside, but she never noticed the shot as she sat staring at the crazy lady dancing in the middle of the emergency room.

Because of that and similar instances, my husband calls me "Doctor Magic," and the name has taken hold with some of my patients.

Children allow us to release the child in ourselves, and part of being a parent as well as a pediatrician is responding to the child within. Through children we rediscover the wonder, delight, and pure joy we often miss as adults. During my fifteen years in pediatrics, I've seen a dismaying trend toward a kind of mechanization of parenting. People forget that having children and rearing them should be filled with joy.

Intellectualizing the parenting experience is like intellectualizing about falling in love. Yes, there are difficult times, scary and frustrating times. I know how tough being a parent can be. It's all on-the-job training, with little or no backup for handling the midnight fever, calming the irritable baby, or juggling job, home, and family. But parenting becomes more difficult if it's treated as though it were something to be mastered like a course in accounting.

A few years ago, on a talk show, a woman called to complain, "I'm twenty-eight years old, I have two children, and I'm finishing graduate school. My three year old glares at me when I have to study. I feel guilty because I'm not spending as much time with my eleven week old as I did with my first child. I have to do schoolwork, wipe up after the cat, answer the phone, and take care of my husband and the household. I feel like a wet noodle."

She summed up with something of an understatement, I thought, "I'm not enjoying my parenting experience."

I told her that she needed to board the cat, buy an answering machine, let her house go to hell a little, and enlist her husband's help with the children and the housework. More important, she had to reevaluate her priorities. She was losing herself in a process rather than enjoying a stage of her life.

Couples need to relax and experience their children. Being a parent is doing the best you can as the kind of person you are. If you develop a natural, easy confidence in yourself, you will transmit this to your child, who will, in turn, feel more secure and loved.

Rearing children is a life activity, like falling in love, getting married, or choosing a career. The best way to approach it is the way you should handle anything in life: gather the necessary basic information, make the best choices you can according to your own values and abilities, then try to enjoy it and get through the difficult times. Child rearing is not something that can or should be graded. And your child is unique, with a temperament and set of responses that are individual and distinct, to which you will have to adapt.

This book will help you to sift through the many choices you face as a parent and to find the ones that work for you. Your needs as a parent have often been ignored or minimized by child-care experts.

One of my patients read that the way to discipline her two-year-old son was to say, "I don't like your behavior, but

I still love you. It's just the way you're behaving that makes me angry." This is perfectly reasonable advice, allowing a parent to discipline a child without threatening the loss of love or self-esteem.

However, as this mother explained to me, "I can't say that. When Jeffrey spills paint on the living-room rug, I'm mad at him, not at his behavior." Just because she read about a way to approach a problem doesn't mean that it will work for her. As long as she shows her love to Jeffrey in countless other ways, she must discipline him in a manner consistent with her feelings.

I have a large pediatric practice which I share with a partner and two associates. Over the years, I've learned that nobody is right all the time. Each doctor in my group makes suggestions to parents based on what seems reasonable at that time, but all babies are different. What works for one family may not work for another.

What is not self-evident is that a parent's instinctive response is usually right. If your child is crying and you feel the urge to pick up the baby, by all means do it. Our complicated world tells us that we must control our feelings. In fact, Freud said that civilization is based on the control of passions. Somehow, love, affection, warmth, and other natural responses have been included in that control. How many times have we heard, "Don't pick up that baby so much—you'll spoil him"?

But there are certain instincts and responses that need not be controlled. Once you have taken the joyful step of having a child, the point is for you to love your baby and introduce your son or daughter to life. We want to raise children who will become happy, secure adults. A child can only achieve that in a household where parents respond, without fear of later consequences, when a baby is tired, bored or unhappy.

Since the Victorian era we have been taught that if something feels good, it's probably bad—everything has its price. That's not true. There are many good things in life without prices attached to them, and one of these is love. You can't structure love, but by responding to your baby's needs, you'll build a foundation for a happy human being.

To be an adequate parent, you must have a certain amount of basic information. I will discuss practical issues such as what to do when your child has a fever and how to make your home safe for a toddler. There are a few absolutes, such as keeping your child in a safe restraint in the car. Beyond that, however, common sense dictates what choices to make. Each parent-child unit is unique. As a parent, you bring to it your twenty or more years of experience, including the way you were parented, and your child brings to it a predetermined set of responses.

You *do* possess the basic qualities you need to be a good parent: love, common sense, and a sense of humor. You can't be perfect, but you can be a "good enough" parent. If you accept that standard, you can forgive your human frailties and relax.

One of my patients had a two year old who wanted to sleep with her parents. Jenny's mother spent a large part of every night putting her back into her own bed. When I asked how she and her husband felt about having Jenny in bed with them, she said that neither of them minded.

"Then why is it a problem for you? Why are you constantly putting Jenny back in her own bed?" I asked.

She answered, "All my friends tell me that you shouldn't have your child in bed with you."

I suggested that Jenny is a very sweet little girl who is somewhat shy and needs a lot of reassurance. I didn't see anything wrong with allowing her that reassurance and comfort in the middle of the night.

Six months later, Jenny's mother told me things were going much better. "Jenny still comes into our bed every night, but she stays in her own bed for longer and longer periods." She used to thrash around a lot, but her parents told her that if she wanted to remain with them she would have to lie quietly.

"So she lies pretty still," said her mother. "But every once in a while in the middle of the night, I'll feel her little hand reach out, and pat my head to be sure I'm there. Then she'll turn over, pat my husband's arm, and go back to sleep."

Those lovely little pats are what being a parent is all about.

LORAINE STERN, M.D.

Los Angeles, 1985

Relax and Enjoy Your Baby

ONE

Your Baby's Doctor

YOU AND YOUR baby's doctor will be seeing a lot of each other during the first two years of your child's life. So it's important that the pediatrician you choose is someone you can trust, someone with whom you feel comfortable. You'll often be seeking guidance from this individual, and good rapport is crucial.

Kindly Dr. Oldendorf may be recommended by everybody on your block, but that doesn't mean Dr. Oldendorf is the right pediatrician for you.

In this chapter, I'll cover how to shop for, interview, and choose your doctor, and what you can expect from the relationship. You should expect your pediatrician to listen attentively to any of your problems about parenting, whether they're marital, medical, or psychological. If your doctor can't help you, he or she should be willing and able to refer you to someone who can.

The ideal way to find a pediatrician is through referral. Your obstetrician may give you the names of pediatricians he or she has worked with and trusts, and may even consider your personality and special needs. The drawback is that sometimes doctors refer you to doctors to whom they're indebted for referrals, so don't rely solely on your obstetrician's recommendation.

Nurses are in an excellent position to evaluate doctors. They know which doctors are competent and compassionate, which ones are readily available and responsive to patients' needs. If you are acquainted with a nurse in the hospital where you plan to have your baby, ask this person for a referral or for his or her opinion of the pediatrician you are considering. Again, this doesn't necessarily mean that the recommendation will be right for you. However, you are likely to get an objective appraisal of one doctor's or several doctors' capabilities.

Some patients have come to me after making a call to the emergency room of their local hospital and asking the nurses on duty for a recommendation. Not all hospitals allow such over-the-transom referrals, however.

You might also phone the department of pediatrics of the medical school near your community and ask for the names of two or three doctors. You are assured, then, that the people you will be considering are associated with a medical school or teaching hospital, which suggests an above-average level of competence and involvement in high-quality medical care.

Your prepared childbirth instructor is another source of

referral. If you feel strongly about breast feeding, members of La Leche will refer you to doctors who are supportive. Local PTAs can also provide help.

Finally, you can even consult the Yellow Pages. Some of my patients have found me simply through the Yellow Pages —they saw a woman's name, and that appealed to them. If that's what you want, the phone book can be a starting point.

After you have a list of names, you'll want to narrow down the list to two or three likely candidates.

Office location is a matter of consideration. The doctor's office should be nearby; if you work far from home, you many want to use two pediatricians: one close to work and a second closer to home. Some of my patients call on the "home" pediatrician for emergencies and acute illnesses at night and on weekends; the doctor near the work location is for scheduled appointments such as checkups that can fit their work schedules.

HOW TO INTERVIEW A PEDIATRICIAN

Make your initial call during the pediatrician's office hours, but, please, not on Monday morning. That's when most pediatric offices are flooded with patient calls from the weekend. Yet no matter what day or time of day you telephone, you should expect a gracious and interested reception.

You might start by stating that you're new in the area or going to have a baby, and are looking for a pediatrician. Wait to see what the response is. Your call may go no further than that because the receptionist may say, "Sorry, but we're not accepting new patients."

However, if the reply indicates that Dr. So-and-So's office

is happy to hear from you, tell the receptionist that you are interested in meeting the doctor.

Secretaries at some offices may say, "The doctor doesn't schedule interviews. Why don't you wait until your baby is sick?" But when you have a real problem is hardly the ideal time to make that first contact. You can't conduct a thoughtful business interview under such conditions. Explain courteously that you can make a better decision when you're not concerned about your baby's well-being, and ask again for an interview. The degree of positive response will give you an idea of how well this office will accommodate your needs and desires.

Some pediatricians will charge for that initial interview, which should last about five or ten minutes. Others will see you at no cost. That should be established during this first phone call.

It's a good idea for the prospective father to attend this interview, too. Fathers are more involved in child care than they used to be, and more and more often it's the father who brings in the infant to see the doctor, especially if working parents really share child care. He should also have the chance to interview and assess the new pediatrician.

Before your interview, you will undoubtedly spend some time in the waiting room, and you can make some valuable observations there. Are there toys for the children to play with? Is there reading material for the parents?

Is the waiting room overcrowded and messy or comfortable and of adequate size? You may hit the office on a bad day and find that a lot of people are waiting. This doesn't necessarily mean that the doctor is overbooked or always running late, but you might ask someone waiting near you if this is a common occurrence. If the response is "We always have to wait two hours," this may not be the office for you. Everybody's time is valuable.

How do the nurses treat the children in the office? Are they understanding and sympathetic? And how do the nurses treat you? Are they efficient and professional, but also warm and pleasant?

Are the staff at the front desk casually talking about patients so you can hear them in the waiting room? You probably don't want your problems discussed within other people's hearing, and that might influence your decision.

You interview a pediatrician for the same reason that you look at a house to see if it's the right one for you. You might fall madly in love with the first doctor at first sight and think it's a waste of time to interview someone else, but you can't make the best choice unless you have a standard of comparison. I'd recommend interviewing at least one other pediatrician.

You should arrive at your interview with a number of questions. Here are some suggestions about questions you should or might ask, but be sure to include anything else that's important to you. The most energetic mother-to-be I ever met had seven typewritten pages of questions. I answered them all, but that's a little excessive, I think.

The first question concerns your doctor's training. Pediatricians should be board-certified or board-eligible, which means they have completed an internship and residency program in pediatrics and have passed or are going to take a special examination for the American Board of Pediatrics.

You will also want to know what the procedure is when the doctor is not on call. No doctor is on call twenty-four hours a day, seven days a week. The doctor may be associated with a group of six or seven other pediatricians who take calls together and cover for each other. Or, as in my practice, two or three partners share the call schedule, so that you won't have to see a strange doctor in an emergency. When your doctor is not on call, you don't want to be referred to the emergency room of a hospital or to a general practitioner. Your own doctor should be available, or you should be able to communicate directly with another pediatrician.

Another useful question is: "How do you feel about phone calls at night?" New parents (and in fact any parent) are usually more concerned about things that happen at night than during the day. You need to determine whether you can reach this doctor easily when you need emergency care or advice.

You can learn about the doctor's attitudes and beliefs by the way he or she answers your questions. For example, if you ask the doctor for an opinion about breast feeding without indicating what your own attitude is, you can soon discover how rigid or flexible this doctor is about a matter of importance to you.

If the pediatrician is condescending and soft-pedals your ideas, prejudices, or concerns, this probably is not the person for you. You won't have the support in child rearing you want. On the other hand, if you are looking to this person for guidance as the expert, and the doctor seems too flippant or glib, you may want to seek elsewhere for the right "fit."

I know one obstetrician who is very cool and easy. He's a terrific doctor and has an informal style. If he's out running when he's paged for an emergency delivery, he'll arrive at the hospital in his jogging shorts. A lot of women love him, but I recently saw a patient who didn't like his relaxed manner. She said, "I had the feeling that whenever I'd ask him a question, he'd answer with a joke. I really needed someone who would give me more authority and make me feel he was taking my questions seriously." So this obstetrician obviously wasn't the right doctor for her.

Whenever you interview a pediatrician, you are entitled to a written fee structure. Before signing on, you should have an indication, not of every possible cost, but of the basics, such as routine office visits and immunizations. Within the community, in private practice, fees among doctors will generally be comparable. They will vary from the higher-income areas (the Beverly Hills or Manhattans) to the suburbs and the inner cities. A word of caution, however. Shopping by price is not a great idea. Lower prices do not necessarily mean better value. Higher prices do not necessarily mean better care. Use your judgment.

Don't forget to discuss the pediatrician's procedures about insurance, and make sure the office accepts your insurance policy. You also want to know if you are responsible for billing your insurance company or if the doctor's office will handle this. These questions can be answered by the doctor's receptionist.

Don't be surprised if you learn that the office accepts credit cards as payment. More and more practices are doing this. It's a reasonable method of payment for both doctor and patient, since the patient has a grace period before payment and the doctor does not have to go through expensive billing procedures which raise the cost of medical care.

In many areas of the country, immunizations can be obtained free at local health clinics, a significant financial saving for patients. However, if your time is limited and time off from work means money, the clinic route may not be worthwhile for you. It may be more economical in the long run to have your child's shots administered at the doctor's office. If you do plan to utilize the facilities of a clinic, you might ask the prospective pediatrician how he or she feels about that arrangement.

In your initial interview, you'll also want to ask about your baby's schedule of visits. Schedules can differ slightly during your child's first year. In our practice, we see an infant at two weeks, at one month, and monthly until six months. We see the baby again at nine months and at one year. In the second year, children come in for checkups at fifteen months, eighteen months, and two years. Visits may be more frequent if the baby was premature or isn't gaining weight well or has some chronic problem.

Finally, after your list of five, seven, or eighty-two questions has been answered by the pediatrician, the one remaining question is: How do the office and doctor make you feel? Do you feel comfortable, valued, and does the doctor listen to you? Or do you feel like part of a large machine? Do you feel at home? Have you found the right atmosphere with the person who will be so close to you and your baby?

When you have covered all the basics, trust your reaction to this person. A good mix between you and your doctor is very important.

Some years ago I knew of a pediatrician in Minnesota whose manner was gruff and brusque. If a mother had to make a repeat visit because her child was still ailing, this man would say, "Well, did you give your son the medicine *exactly* the way I told you to?"

The mother would say, "Yes," after which he would ask, "Did you miss any doses at all?"

Of course, people are likely to miss doses. But this doctor would always find a way to imply that it was the mother's fault. Surprisingly enough, women *flocked* to this guy despite his manner. He was a good doctor, I might add.

Some people need firm direction from their doctors. Others need someone who is loose, who respects the way they live and how they want to rear their child. An evaluation from a nurse or a friend may not take your particular needs into account. When you meet the doctor yourself, you can make your own evaluation according to what you expect and need.

THE PSYCHOLOGICAL ROLE OF THE PEDIATRICIAN

When asked if I deal with psychological issues in my practice, my answer is: "Yes, but only eighty or ninety percent of the time."

I'm not trying to wear two hats, but one primary role of the pediatrician is that of psychologist. Fortunately, we no longer live in a society where polio epidemics are rampant and where many life-endangering diseases routinely threaten children's lives. So I have many opportunities to listen to my patients' problems, and if I can't help them directly, I'll refer them to the person who can. I've been a marriage counselor, a social director, an emotional support, and a "shoulder to cry on" on many occasions.

As the years go by, I've come to believe that the pediatrician's major responsibility is to relieve parental anxiety. My patients are usually surprised by this. They think of doctors as exalted beings who are preoccupied with arcane information and sophisticated equipment, as people who tell them what to do. They're not used to concern, which is what we *should* be best at offering. My colleagues and I receive a lot of mail from grateful parents who are amazed at the support they receive from us. Actually, parents should *expect* this.

Some mothers will feel apologetic about bringing in a child for what is diagnosed as "just" a common cold. I always try to let them know that I'm glad they brought in their child. There's nothing wrong with coming in with what is proved to be a minor illness. Sometimes it's not, and your visits to your doctor are a learning experience.

Equally important, as a recent study showed, parents who make repeated visits to a pediatrician with seemingly insignificant concerns are often fearful of something else. For example, if a mother frequently brings in her healthy two year old with minor problems, I might, in questioning the woman, discover that she had a sister who died of leukemia and is terrified that the disease will strike her child. If I can uncover the underlying anxiety, I can then address it and help my patient allay her fears or refer her to someone who can.

Pediatricians *want* to help parents—especially new parents—get through their child's first few years successfully. While doctors are generally very busy (like anyone else), you shouldn't be reluctant to call if you have a problem or anticipate that your call will be resented. A mother may preface a call by saying "I know you're very busy, but . . . " and will act as though she's unworthy of taking up my time. I always reassure her that I'm busy with *patients,* and when you're a patient, you have a right to call. Your baby's doctor is there to help you.

At least five times a day a parent will say to me, "This is a really dumb question, but . . . " And those are always the *best* questions. The only dumb question is the one you're afraid to ask. That question may be about something you really had no way of knowing and should have asked. Or it could have been that you were concerned about a potential problem and needed reassurance. One of my mothers came in with her baby on a Monday, having spent the entire weekend unable to eat or sleep. She thought a minor bump on her child's head was the same problem as her friend's baby had with a congenital malformation of the brain. I could have told her over the phone that it wasn't anything at all, and she wouldn't have had to put herself through all that anguish.

I try to offer my patients not only the best medical advice, but something intangible that's related to my role as a doctor. A framed quote that hangs on the wall of my office sums it up. I came across the quote in a medical article and found it so moving that I told my husband about it. He was touched as well and had the fifteenth-century saying set in type for me. The role of the doctor, the saying reads, is

> To cure sometimes
> to relieve often
> to comfort always.

TWO

That Magic Moment: Delivery

IN ONE OF my favorite cartoon strips, "Cathy" by Cathy Guisewhite, two women in an office are talking about an impending birth. Some fellows who are listening ask each other, "How could you consider a home birth now that the hospital has a birthing room?" another young man asks, "Are you guys doing Lamaze or Leboyer?" and another, "Ruth and I are doing Lamaze and yoga," while a mustachioed man adds, "We're into classical music for the unborn."

The cartoon closes with Cathy's fiftyish boss asking her, "Whatever happened to the good old days when women were the only ones who got pregnant?"

Not only does the cartoon illustrate the involvement of

men in the birth process and the number of options available to couples, but also that people are often dogmatic about the right way to have a baby.

There is no "right way." Women can have their babies using the Bradley or Lamaze method or with yoga, in a university hospital or a community hospital, lying down or squatting. The best method is the one that feels best and makes good medical sense. Whether or not you want to have completely natural childbirth or use some pain relief, whether or not the baby's father will be with you for delivery are choices that you as a couple should make in concert with your obstetrician.

LAMAZE- AND BRADLEY-PREPARED CHILDBIRTH

Most prepared childbirth classes use the techniques of Lamaze or Bradley or the instructor's own combination of the two. Both methods are based on the same principle: women who understand labor and become participants in controlling and facilitating the process will have less pain and shorter labors and deliver healthier babies. The experience of labor then becomes not a period of suffering that must be endured but a joyful process that a woman can master.

Lamaze developed his techniques in the late 1950s and emphasizes breathing and relaxation exercises. Bradley's method is different, but his major contribution, which all programs have now adopted, was the participation of the father.

Bradley's idea to include the father came about, as he describes in his book *Husband Coached Childbirth,* when he had attended a childbirth-trained mother's delivery. Afterward, he leaned over the table to shake her hand and congratulate her, as was his custom. The young mother exuberantly kissed him, exclaiming happily, "Thank you for showing me how!" It later struck him: What was this lovely woman kissing *him* for while her husband sat uselessly in the waiting room? He says, "I am not the least bit interested in having my patients fall in love with me, but I feel deeply the responsibility, as an obstetrician, to see that the act of bearing a child makes them fall more in love with the father of the baby."

That's the philosophy that began Bradley's crusade for husband-coached childbirth, and now, twenty years later, virtually all childbirth education programs include fathers.

A patient of mine who's also the wife of an obstetrician decided, simply out of curiosity, to take Lamaze training for her first baby and Bradley for the second. She felt that both were equally effective but that the Lamaze course gave more specific instructions while the Bradley technique allowed the parents to develop their specific personal techniques based on their own personalities and their own relationship.

Prepared childbirth classes also include information about the newborn and postpartum adjustment, both physical and emotional. The birth center in which I participate has a twelve-week course, with six or eight classes devoted to the traditional childbirth training. The rest cover everything from breast feeding to preparation for possible cesarean section.

Prepared childbirth classes can give parents an additional benefit: after spending many weeks with the same people, all of whom will have babies at about the same time, friendships develop which often continue. Class members become a kind of extended family, and parents keep in touch with each other to share experiences and support each other.

The essence of "natural" childbirth is that it should be as easy and simple as possible. Several years ago some women, especially in California, were delivering babies underwater in spas and hot tubs, and *Time* magazine had a good time covering this transient phenomenon. This somewhat bizarre trend began when a French obstetrician realized that women in labor in hospitals are not as relaxed as they would be at home, and he wanted to increase their relaxation in order to speed labor along. He asked some women who were about to give birth to submerge themselves in a warm bath for its well-known soothing effect. Often, however, the women relaxed so completely that their babies were precipitously born in the tub. This submersion was not intended to be a birthing technique, but a means for relaxing mothers and shortening labor. Having a baby underwater is a cumbersome and impractical idea.

While natural-childbirth followers do not advocate pain relief with medication, emphasizing that mothers should be helped to deal with pain so that medication is not necessary, a long labor with a tired mother can, on some occasions, be facilitated with a mild relaxant. The whole point of natural childbirth is to have a healthy baby and a healthy and fulfilled mother, and if a mild relaxant can help to avoid a cesarean section or undue fatigue, it's not a failure of natural childbirth but common sense to take advantage of it.

CESAREAN SECTIONS

One in four or five women who deliver in a hospital will require a cesarean section, which means that the baby is delivered through a surgical incision in the lower abdomen. The reasons are many: labor is not progressing; the baby shows signs of not tolerating labor well; the mother develops a medical problem; or the mother has herpes lesions. Most birth centers and prepared childbirth classes devote a session to cesarean section so that the father can be present to accompany the mother and witness the birth of his baby. Indeed, under these circumstances, the father becomes even more important to the baby. Mothers are able to hold and look at their babies immediately after birth if they have had a spinal anesthesia and are awake, but they can't do very much else since they're immobilized on the operating table. The father then becomes the primary person to introduce his child to the world and accompany the baby to the nursery while the mother recovers.

We must not forget, however, that a mother's labor coach and companion for delivery, whether vaginal or cesarean, need not always be the father. Over the years I've attended many births where a sister or friend of the mother's was the labor coach, or where father attended mother until the C-section but stopped at the door to the operating room. The couples had come to an understanding about this beforehand, and each woman told me that she would have preferred to have her husband with her, but only if he'd wanted to.

Remember that the experience of childbirth is not an end in itself but a means for delivering a healthy baby to a healthy mother. Each labor is different, and each woman is different. Whatever your fantasies or expectations, if you have confidence in your obstetrician, this support will ensure a positive experience and a good, healthy baby.

THE WAYS OF NEWBORNS

Mothers are delighted and excited when they hear their newborn's first cry. But Dr. Frederick Leboyer believed that this was a cry of pain, a response to the stress of the birth process and the child's emergence into a harsh, cold world.

He looked at childbirth from a baby's point of view and developed a method of delivery designed to make gentler the transition from a buoyant, warm, water-filled womb into the cold, noisy, brightly lit delivery room.

He surmised that a warm bath might duplicate the child's feelings of being in the water-filled amniotic sac and help the infant to relax. With his technique, the father lowers the baby into warm water, allowing the arms and legs to move freely, and then gradually lifts the baby out of the water and into the air. This bath is not intended for cleansing, but to ease the transition from the water-filled world the infant has known to a totally new environment. During delivery, the father has mainly been an observer and supporter, but now he has a chance to play an active role and to have time alone with the baby. Some babies will cry anyway, but many will relax blissfully in the bath, stare intently at their fathers, and a few will even smile, while their fathers hold and stroke them in the warm water.

Not all hospitals currently offer the Leboyer bath. In my opinion, it's a lovely procedure and I wish all hospitals had it as a routine part of delivery.

In almost all hospitals, an antibiotic ointment is instilled in a baby's eyes shortly after birth. Formerly, silver nitrate drops were used; but not only do they produce significant irritation, they are not effective against the most common cause of newborn eye infection—an organism called chlamydia.

Newborns also receive an injection of vitamin K. This prevents a rare but serious disorder called "hemorrhagic disease of the newborn," to which breast-fed babies are particularly prone. There are no side effects to the injection, and all babies should have it.

After the umbilical cord is clamped, many nurseries apply

a blue dye to the stump, which acts as an antibacterial coating.

Most states require a blood test before the baby leaves the hospital. This is a screening test for some metabolic disorders that can cause mental retardation if not diagnosed early. It requires just a few drops of blood from the baby's foot.

People frequently ask if newborns can see. Anyone who has been stared at intently by a newborn cannot possibly entertain this thought. Newborns can't read freeway signs at two hundred feet, but an ideal focal length in the first weeks is about eighteen inches, or the distance from breast to mother's face—the only distance a baby needs to see. Since newborns are a little nearsighted, seeing things better up close, they may look at their noses a lot and appear cross-eyed. If that happens occasionally, it's normal. You will discover that newborns are not just little bundles of primitive reflexes, but are complicated beings who see, smell, taste, hear, feel, and have definite preferences.

Babies' most obvious form of communication is crying, and parents quickly learn to distinguish among the "I'm hungry" wail, the "I'm bored" cry, and the "I'm wet and want to be changed" whimper. But there are more subtle ways that babies communicate. Having examined a newborn in the nursery, I went to the mother's room to tell her how healthy and beautiful her baby was. The nurses had put a shirt on her baby with long cuffs to cover his hands because he was scratching his face with his fingernails. The father said, "I don't think he likes to have his hands covered," and indeed, he was right. When the baby's hands were covered he was agitated and unhappy, and once his hands were free, he relaxed. This father, who had had no previous experience with infants, paid attention to his baby's responses to learn about his baby.

When babies are startled, they produce a "Moro reflex" —they jerk, extend their arms, then bring their hands together with their eyes wide open in surprise. Your baby may have this response to a soft noise such as the phone ringing. This is your assurance that the baby can hear normally. A baby may also demonstrate hearing by pausing in movement as if listening when a noise occurs. One day, as I was examining a baby by myself in a big, empty nursery, a housekeeper was quietly washing the floor in another room. The baby and I were gazing at each other in a lovely moment of silent communication when she suddenly jumped with what appeared to be a spontaneous Moro's reflex.

What startled this baby? I wondered. Was it a gas bubble, or did something startle her as she was falling asleep? When it happened again, I realized that way off in the other room the housekeeper made a slight sound whenever she put her mop in the bucket. The baby, demonstrating a poignant sensitivity, was responding to a sound that I could barely hear.

In the movie *The Amazing Newborn,* a mother talks to her child in familiar repetitive baby talk. While she says "Pretty baby, oh, what a pretty baby" over and over, the baby moves in an apparently random way. The film and soundtrack are then slowed down so that the mother sounds like Smoky the Bear, speaking v-e-rrrrry slowly. It then becomes obvious that the baby's movements are not only graceful, but completely in time with the mother's sounds and the rhythm of her voice. The baby is acting as an orchestra, with the mother as conductor.

If you pick babies up by their hands, their heads will flop backward, but when they are on their stomachs, they can lift their heads and turn them from side to side. This reassures us that newborns can breathe easily when face down lying on their stomachs.

There is also the "quiet alert state," when hunger, diaper changing, and the need for sleep have all been satisfied. During this period, the baby has a chance to look around and observe the world. Take advantage of these times to play with your newborn, even if the dishes need washing.

Newborns soon learn to imitate their parents' facial expressions. This is the time when parents have a lot of fun playing face-making games.

The first smile that we see on a baby's face is an egocentric one, signifying internal contentment and comfort. It's not because of gas, as many people would have it, but it's also not because of any social interaction. On the other hand, the first time a child smiles in response to a human face, usually the mother's, is a monumental event. This is the first evidence that the baby can see relationships—"The person I see is connected with a good feeling, and therefore this person's face makes me feel good." This is how an infant first learns to love, the basis for all relationships later in life.

If you hold your newborn upright, feet flat on a table top, and move the baby forward, the feet and legs will move as if the baby is walking. This is a primitive reflex that disappears soon and reappears when it is time to walk.

In the first months of life there are times when a baby needs to cry just to release pent-up tension. The infant has left the warm, dark, comfortable environment of the womb for a harsh, dissonant, stressful world of light and sound. If you try everything to comfort the child and nothing helps, realize that you also may have experienced this in your first weeks after delivery. New mothers often have the feeling that they just need a good cry to release their emotions. If the baby needs the same release, maybe you can even cry together.

Your infant's responses are unique to your relationship with him or her, and as the two of you become acquainted, you will discover what makes your baby distinctive and what sort of person you will be living with.

Jaundice of the Newborn

During the first few days of life, many infants become jaundiced, which means that their skin and the whites of their eyes turn yellow because of a substance called bilirubin, produced by the breakdown of excess red blood cells with which all babies are born. Jaundice can be the result of a minor blood incompatibility between baby and mother, but most often it's what we call *idiopathic* or *physiologic,* which are fancy words that mean "we don't know what causes it, but it isn't anything bad."

Ten percent of normal babies will develop jaundice by the second or third day of life. Babies who stay only one or two days in the hospital need to be checked in the pediatrician's office in a day or two to make sure this hasn't developed after they leave the nursery. Jaundice in and of itself is not abnormal, and it's rare that the level of bilirubin can rise far enough to be toxic to the baby's brain.

Treatment is preventive, administered before the jaundice reaches a worrisome level, and the treatment is simple. When I was an intern at UCLA, there was a wonderful Polish nurse in the nursery who seemed ancient to me at the time, although she was probably all of fifty. She said that when she put the babies near the window, their jaundice decreased. At the time, I thought that was nothing but folk medicine, but shortly thereafter there was scientific confirmation of the fact that there is a wave length of light present in both sunlight and fluorescent light that breaks bilirubin down into a harmless substance that babies can easily excrete.

Phototherapy, or the use of light for lowering jaundice, has been around for fifteen or twenty years and doesn't appear to have any long-term consequences. The baby is placed under a bank of fluorescent lights in just a diaper or nude, with a cover over the eyes. The bulk of the day, with time out for feeding and visiting, is spent under the light. The bilirubin level is checked at intervals via a little blood drawn from the infant's heel.

Jaundice may prolong a baby's hospital stay by a day or two, and to avoid that some pediatricians use a program of at home phototherapy in which a unit of lights can be rented from a local pharmacy or hospital to treat the baby. In many ways, this is better than having the baby stay in the hospital, for baby and parents are not separated and hospital bills aren't mounting up. However, there are drawbacks. The baby must have a constant attendant twenty-four hours a day, which can be difficult if there aren't several people to take responsibility and alternate three- or four-hour shifts. The baby's temperature as well as the ambient temperature must be constantly monitored, the mask has to be checked to be sure it hasn't slipped off, and the baby must be given frequent feedings of water in between regular breast or bottle feedings. The baby also must be seen at least daily in the pediatrician's office.

Since this is a time when parents may be tired and overwhelmed by the excitement of new parenthood, the additional unfamiliar, demanding routine may be more stressful than letting the baby stay in the hospital and getting it over with.

Jaundice usually disappears after a few days, but sometimes a baby has persistent mild jaundice for several weeks. Some doctors tell mothers to stop nursing, but there's no need for that. Formula feeding for twenty-four hours, while pumping your breasts to maintain milk flow, is usually enough to drop the bilirubin level. No one knows why this works, but you should resume nursing as soon as the bilirubin level is down.

Other Minor Problems

Many babies are born with swollen breasts, which may even discharge a little milky fluid. A useless but interesting piece of trivia is that this milk, thought to have magical properties in bygone days, was known as witches' milk and was collected for use in potions. The swelling goes away in a few weeks, but if the area becomes red, consult your pediatrician immediately, for this tissue can, in rare cases, become infected.

At about three to five days, some female babies may produce a little bright red blood in their diaper. This normal phenomenon, called "withdrawal bleeding," is something like a period, caused by the decreasing levels of the mother's pregnancy hormones, the same hormones that cause breast enlargement. Consider it a good sign, for you now have evidence that your little girl has a uterus that will function in the future.

From a few days to a few weeks of age, a white coating may appear on the baby's tongue that looks like curds of milk. This is called thrush, a fungal infection that probably occurs because babies suck so vigorously that they irritate the inside of their mouth. It doesn't hurt, but when we find it we treat it with medicine applied topically to the membranes in the mouth after the baby has eaten. Sometimes it takes three or four weeks and several refills of medication to clear up a thrush infection.

A rash, sometimes called a "flea-bite rash," can occur in

the first week. I recently realized that I shouldn't refer to it as "flea bite" because one of my mothers went home and fumigated her house. A flea-bite rash does resemble small insect bites, but it has nothing to do with bugs. It goes away by itself after a few days.

Little white dots may appear on the baby's nose right after birth. Sometimes the dots involve the cheeks and forehead. These are called "milia" and are the result of blocked oil glands. These, too, will go away by themselves.

As to birthmarks, most are not present at birth but develop later, despite their name. One kind that is present at birth is called a flame nevus, which some people call a "stork bite." These are flat, reddish, flamelike marks on the back of the neck, the forehead, and the eyelids. They go away in the first year.

Mongolian spots have nothing to do with being mongoloid or with Down's syndrome, but occur in dark-complexioned babies as a gray-blue flat discoloration near the tail bone and can be one large mark or a collection of smaller ones. This mark also usually disappears in the first few years but, due to its location, is rarely a cosmetic problem.

CIRCUMCISION: THE UNKINDEST CUT

If your baby is a boy, you will be asked if you want him circumcised—the flap of skin at the end of the penis removed. The act of asking this question of a parent implies that the procedure is, to a certain extent, desirable. I believe that routine circumcision of the newborn is, as Shakespeare said in another context, the "unkindest cut of all." It is not only unkind, but painful, unnecessary, and dangerous.

About eight years ago the American Academy of Pediatrics and the American College of Obstetrics published statements saying that routine neonatal circumcision is unnecessary and that the risks outweigh the benefits, but obstetricians and the general public have largely ignored these statements. Studies have shown that educating parents about the risks of circumcision has little effect on their behavior, and the majority still have their boys circumcised. The reasons for doing so are vague: "Everybody does it," "It's cleaner," or "I thought it was necessary" are the usual parental responses. In a study at the University of Utah, pediatrician Dr. Lucy Osborne asked parents why they had their baby boys circumcised, and 14 percent of them had *no reason!* Obviously, ritual circumcision—for example, the Jewish ceremonial *bris* —is a different issue. The choice of having it done is religious, and the arguments for and against are largely nonmedical.

Circumcision is the most commonly performed surgical procedure in the United States; while 85 to 90 percent of American males are circumcised, 85 to 90 percent of males in the rest of the world are not. There's an old saying: "Fifty million Frenchmen can't be wrong." If we're doing something the rest of the world isn't doing, we must examine whether there's a good reason for us to continue the practice.

In the Victorian era, routine neonatal circumcision was popular because it was thought that circumcising the newborn would prevent "hypersexuality" later and would keep children from masturbating (then considered an unhealthy practice). In addition, it was believed that circumcision could alleviate or prevent illnesses ranging from rheumatism to indigestion. Of course, this is nonsense.

In that era, the practice of circumcision increased throughout the world and then gradually declined over the next fifty years everywhere except in the United States. By the 1980s, the procedure is hardly performed in Europe at all, although it's just as commonplace here as it ever was.

Parents may think that if their son is not circumcised, he will seem an outsider later, particularly in the locker room. While it's true that most boys are circumcised, it is important to understand that the boy who is not circumcised is as normal as the other boys who have been altered. In a similar vein, some people believe that if a father is circumcised, his son should be, too. In his book *Circumcision, a Health Fallacy,* Edward Wallerstein, an advocate of leaving male anatomy alone, tells of a circumcised father with an uncircumcised son. At around age three, the child asked his father about the difference between them. The father told the son, "When I was a baby, they thought it was a good idea to cut off that part of the penis."

The son thought for a minute and then said, "That was sure dumb," and that was the end of it.

The myth that circumcision reduces the risk of cancer of the penis in the male and cancer of the cervix in the female is untrue. There is no evidence that uncircumcised men contract penile cancer more frequently than circumcised men. Jewish women whose husbands are circumcised have a lower rate of cervical cancer than non-Jewish women whose husbands are not circumcised, so people came to believe that circumcision prevented cancer of the cervix. But in recent years we've discovered that there are genetic predispositions to certain forms of cancer. The fact that Jewish males are circumcised does not account for the low rate of cervical cancer. It's just that Jewish women are less genetically inclined to develop cervical cancer. Conversely, there is a rise in cervical cancer among teenaged girls who are sexually active, and most of their partners are circumcised.

Another fallacy is that the man who has been circumcised has more sexual "staying power," can remain erect longer and has greater sexual prowess. Totally false. In fact, premature ejaculation is the most common complaint of men seeking treatment for sexual dysfunction, and most of them are circumcised.

There is also the assumption that a circumcised penis is cleaner. There is a secretion under the foreskin called smegma, which is normal and similar to mucus. It's true that boys without foreskins don't have these secretions, but that doesn't mean that the foreskin is unclean. It was once believed that uncircumcised males were more susceptible to venereal disease, that germs could collect underneath the foreskin. There's no evidence that circumcision lessens the risk of venereal disease.

The only advice necessary for taking care of the foreskin is to wash it with the same attention to hygiene given to any other part of the body. There's nothing scary or complicated about the uncircumcised penis. As Dr. Alex Comfort said, "Wash, don't amputate." I've heard of many boys who were circumcised because a poorly informed doctor thought that the foreskin was too tight when it couldn't be pulled back. Foreskins don't retract in babies; that's just the way they're made. Only after three to five years can they be pulled back even halfway.

The foreskin was put there for a purpose. It protects the opening at the end of the penis, the meatus, through which males urinate. Boys who no longer have this protection often develop ulcers around the meatus, which can lead to later narrowing of the opening and problems with urination.

Another argument has it that if your son is not circumcised at birth, he may need the operation later. The rate of neonatal circumcision in Finland is almost zero, and the rate among older men is about 6 in 100,000. In other words, the chances are very small that adult circumcision will be necessary; and even if it is, adults are better able to tolerate complications such as infection and bleeding than are newborns.

Two to four percent of circumcised males develop infections, and while most of these are minor and of little concern, some can be serious. That makes sense, since the fresh wound is immediately enclosed in a diaper into which the infant urinates and defecates, not the best environment for clean wound healing. Normal infants can bleed from the circumcision site, and babies with unsuspected bleeding disorders can develop a serious problem.

Some people think that circumcision doesn't hurt. Anyone who has been present when a clamp was placed on a newborn's foreskin can never again doubt that the procedure hurts. An infant who's just gone through the stress of birth should emerge into a world that's loving and tender. Why should we immediately attack his most precious possession?

One day I attended, with one of my obstetrical colleagues, a natural birth with soft lights, a quiet room, a Leboyer bath, all things kind and gentle. A few minutes later the obstetrician came into the nursery to circumcise another newborn. This baby boy was lying on a table tied to a little board with his penis poking through a sterile drape.

As the doctor was getting ready to apply the clamp, I asked, "How can you do this after that lovely, warm delivery?"

His reply was "Don't ask."

A strange thing about circumcision is this: for any other operation, the surgeon who performs the procedure would follow the patient's progress in the hospital and take care of any later complications. Circumcision is traditionally performed by obstetricians, who almost never see the patient again. Pediatricians see the complications and deal with the problems, and, therefore, most obstetricians think that circumcision is a benign uncomplicated procedure and don't inform parents about the negative aspects.

Any surgical procedure should be undertaken only after "informed consent," which means that the patient or the patient's guardian is fully aware of the benefits and the risks —and the benefits, of course, should outweigh the risks.

The natural-childbirth movement and the humanization of birth practices arose when public awareness and pressure met with the cooperation of the medical community. Since the medical establishment has been remiss, I hope someday a public action group will effectively discourage circumcision.

BONDING

The term *bonding* has become a catchword lately. Many of my patients have heard or read a great deal about the importance of bonding and are determined to do it "the right way." Before deciding whether or not there *is* a right way, I'd like to talk about what bonding means.

Bonding is the process by which parents and newborn babies fall in love with each other. Specifically it refers to that intense interaction that occurs immediately after birth between mother and child (we also recognize the importance of father/newborn bonding as well). Ideally, bonding is the formation of a profound attachment which begins early in life and develops over the period of a lifetime.

Some parents fall in love with their infants immediately after birth. For others the process may take hours or even days. Just as the emotion of love is a distinct experience for each person, so bonding, or attachment to your baby, is unique. It is affected by the mother's psychological history, the quality of parenting in her own childhood, and her relationship with the father of her child.

Our understanding of the nature and importance of bonding comes from the studies of pediatricians Marshall Klaus and John Kennell at Case Western Reserve University in Ohio. In the 1970s, they studied the attachment behavior and attitudes of mothers who were separated from their babies shortly after birth.

Because these babies were small or premature or in poor health at birth, they were immediately placed in special nurseries known as neonatal intensive care units. Isolated from the warmth and intimacy of contact with their parents, the newborns depended on tubes, catheters, and intravenous feeding for survival. Mothers and fathers were excluded from the neonatal ICUs because of fear of infection, later discovered to be unfounded. When they did visit, they could only view their babies through the nursery window.

It was necessary for some of these infants to spend months in the nursery. When they were finally allowed to join their parents, a surprising thing happened. Over time, the researchers discovered that these children were returning to the medical system more frequently than other children—not only for health problems but for evidence of neglect and physical abuse.

The researchers proposed that there was a critical process during the newborn period that failed to take hold in these families, and the scientists related it to the early separation between mothers and babies. Klaus and Kennell's initial studies involved only mothers and their healthy newborns in the postnatal period. They asked the mothers to fill out questionnaires, conducted interviews with them, and observed their actions.

It was found that the women's attitudes toward their babies and their feelings of adequacy as mothers in subsequent weeks varied according to the mothers' experience in the first minutes, hours, and days of the babies' life.

Klaus and Kennell also found that there was a consistent and predictable pattern of touching, stroking, and eye contact that occurred between mothers and newborns. All mothers and infants behave in almost the same way. For example, the mother starts by gently touching the baby's finger with her finger. She then holds the baby's hand, and strokes the baby with her fingertips and hands. Both father and mother will hold the baby so that they are face to face, looking each other in the eye. They will croon to the baby softly and lovingly.

Those women who had plenty of time with their newborns, who were able to touch and talk to their babies for as long as they wanted, had more positive feelings toward the infants and their own motherhood than those who were deprived of this experience. In one study the researchers found that a period of contact as short as five minutes after birth made a positive difference in the mother's attachment to her baby.

What happens during this critical period of attachment? For one thing, the parents are now actually experiencing the person about whom they have fantasized for nine months. This child is now a "reality" and a part of the outside world, and inevitably differs from the child that they envisioned when he or she was *in utero.* There is no way that this baby could possibly be exactly as imagined. I am not talking about having a boy instead of a girl or a brunette instead of a blonde, but about other aspects of personality and temperament that might be unexpected (such as having a very active baby when you expected a placid one).

For most parents, when they look at their new baby, there is acceptance of the uniqueness and individuality of this new person. This is often accompanied by feelings of joy and wonder. Also, the baby gazes back at the parents. This intense contact is a profound experience for both the parents and the child. When parents first see their baby and the child's eyes are closed, they will frequently say things like "Open your eyes so I know you're alive!" or "Here I am—I'm your mommy, look at me!"

As we all know, newborns spend a lot of time sleeping, crying, or eating. Yet there are periods when they are in what is known as a quiet-alert state, during which they look around and are obviously feeling physically comfortable. These periods normally last only from ten seconds to five minutes. But immediately after birth, many babies can spend up to an hour in this state. In fact a baby may spend a longer times in the quiet-alert state immediately after birth than ever again in the first few weeks of life.

During this time, babies look very intensely at the people looking at them—a moving experience for any adult. This eye contact is the first time that parents experience a response from their baby as another human being.

Parents also need to touch and feel the baby, and to count fingers and toes to make sure everything is accounted for. Some anxiety about having a healthy, normal baby is natural for all parents. The touching, stroking, and finger counting are extremely reassuring for the parents as well as pleasurable for the baby.

These behaviors are not things that you need to think about or that you will do because you read about them here. They are spontaneous human reactions to a significant life event.

With so much going on, what happens if this critical period of attachment is interrupted?

In their initial research, Klaus and Kennell concluded that if there were no opportunity for the bonding process immediately after delivery, there would be no second chance—it was now or never. There would be negative effects for the future growth and development of this parent-child relationship, and further change was not possible. Their research was highly publicized and caused parents to believe that if this period were interrupted, all was lost. People became frantic about disrupting early moments of bonding, and the result was an unfortunate overreaction.

Klaus and Kennell have subsequently modified their previous studies, but this new work hasn't received such widespread publicity. In *Parent-Infant Bonding,* the 1982 revised edition of their 1976 book *Maternal-Infant Bonding,* the researchers again state that, if possible, the parents' privacy and contact with their babies right after birth should be respected. Nevertheless, bonding is a continuing complex process. There is no reason why, say Klaus and Kennell, having been interrupted, attachment between the mother, the father, and the child cannot proceed beautifully and profoundly, even if it is begun after the critical period.

The perspective we now have on bonding and on the immediate newborn period is that it *is* an important time. Everything should be done so that parents and babies can have a private time immediately after birth without interference from hospital staff and away from the clattering of bedpans.

However, there are times when the bonding period will have to be interrupted. Babies are sometimes born with problems that must be tended to immediately after birth.

They may have to be transferred to a neonatal intensive care unit, often in another hospital. The mother may also have experienced problems during childbirth, and she may not be ready for involvement with her infant immediately after delivery.

If your bonding process is interrupted for any reason, this doesn't mean that you will not be able to love your baby properly. Nor does it mean that your child will fail to love you. Dr. Stella Chess, child psychiatrist at the New York University School of Medicine, recently stressed that the absence of the bonding period need not doom the infant to less than optimal development. If a mother's bonding with her baby is impaired, this will not necessarily affect the child's later emotional relationships, Dr. Chess maintains.

If your bonding is interrupted, what can you do?

The good news is that bonding proceeds with the father as well as with the mother. The father can hold the baby immediately after birth, give the infant the Leboyer bath, and hold the baby in the nursery until mother and infant can be reunited.

If your newborn must be transferred to a neonatal ICU in another hospital, you can ask to be transferred with your baby. It this is not possible, the father should accompany the baby to the ICU and should spend as much time there as possible until you are able to visit.

Recently I was involved in a birth in which the infant was small and ailing. It's good medical practice, even if babies are only slightly ill, to treat the illness seriously and intensively until the newborns are completely well. This baby was to be transferred to a neonatal ICU for a day or two.

I went into the delivery room to talk with the mother, and the patient's obstetrician was in the room. The mother asked him whether he thought she should be transferred along with the infant. The obstetrician's reply was, "Yes, I believe in bonding."

Although I was pleased that he was sensitive to the importance of mother and infant being together, I was struck by the detachment in his voice. Bonding isn't like a religion, something to "believe in," but the most natural thing in the world—falling in love when you first become acquainted with your newborn child. It should be seen for the spontaneous experience it is. Often nurses will write in their notes, "Baby out to mother for bonding," as though they were ordering a performance, "Okay—bond."

Still and all, the medical establishment is now aware that newborn babies and parents need time alone to communicate with each other. Because of Klaus and Kennell's work, mothers and fathers of babies who are placed in neonatal ICUs are encouraged to visit any time of the day or night and to spend as much time as they want with their infants. If the baby is not breast-feeding or cannot be held all the time, parents are at least given the opportunity to be close to their child in whatever way is possible.

As with all relationships, bonding develops and changes over time. We should not become compulsive about making a normal life process into a complicated task to master. If the moments after birth were not exactly what you hoped they would be, you still have many days, months and years ahead of you to love your child.

It's also helpful to realize that bonding occurs at different rates and times in various individuals. At first, some parents have the experience of not feeling connected to their babies. They feel numb and confused because the event of birth itself is so overwhelming.

Other factors in the parents' life can also influence their reaction to their baby. A geographic move, especially away from their family, a job change, marriage difficulties, or financial problems can all affect their emotional response to their newborn child. Some people need a longer time to adjust, and during that time some mothers don't have the comfortable, loving feelings toward their baby that they expected to have. Perhaps as many as 8 to 10 percent of women feel depressed following delivery for a week or two, sometimes for physical reasons but often just because of a normal human reaction to a profound life experience.

Women who feel let-down may blame themselves and fear they will be inadequate mothers. Here the support of the child's father is critical. If he can be especially loving, attentive, and patient, he can help alleviate the new mother's distress. And the mother will be more likely to get through this transition with feelings of self-esteem and adequacy intact.

While it's important to share your confusion and depressive thoughts with your mate, it's equally important that he not feel he has to do something to make it all right. This is not the time for him to take charge. What counts is that he listens and understands your feelings.

If you feel you're having difficulty relating to your baby, don't be embarrassed to speak to your pediatrician or to the nurses on the obstetric floor. Doctors and nurses have all dealt with these reactions in new mothers. They can bring in an appropriate counselor, if necessary, or at least discuss your feelings with you to help you through the confusion. It doesn't mean you're neurotic or a bad mother or certifiably crazy.

It's normal to feel confused, overwhelmed, or numb. Your own inner tumult has to subside before you can adjust to the new feelings that being a parent arouses, and if you allow yourself to adjust as slowly as you need, your feelings will sort themselves out in a short time.

Finally, your emotional response will be influenced by the personality of your newborn—that very active participant in the parent-child relationship. Your child has a personality even before birth and generally enters the world in his or her unique way.

One weekend, when I was on call, I saw just how different and special each child can be.

Three cesarean sections took place in a twelve-hour period, all performed by the same obstetrician in the same delivery room. The three young women were all first-time mothers, and their babies were all in breech position. The fathers were present, there was a Leboyer bath for each delivery, and the lights were dim. And all the babies turned out to be girls! It was as ideal a situation as could be for an observer of human behavior. None of the babies was in distress, and all of the mothers were healthy.

The first baby cried the instant she hit the air and went on crying unless she was held very close. In the bath she screamed, under the warmer she screamed, when her mother held her she screamed. Nothing helped until she rested for a while in the nursery. The second baby cried lustily for a minute, then looked around, cried, looked around, and repeated the pattern as long as I was in the delivery room. When the obstetrician delivered the third baby, he said, "She looks surprised." Her mouth was shaped in an "O," and she never stopped gazing around her. On her face was a look of wonder, as if she were saying, "What in the world is going on here?" When you looked at her, she looked back at you.

Each of the babies, delivered under very similar circumstances, demonstrated her own particular personality and way of reacting to the world, even during her first few minutes of life! Each one, very likely, affected the kind of relationship she will have with her parents. Babies who look at their parents very deeply and interact easily elicit different responses from babies who look away or are more self-absorbed.

The importance of what we've been discussing is this: the first contact between parents and infants is a powerful and important time. People are fortunate if that contact meets all their expectations and early bonding occurs.

For others, however, that time doesn't go smoothly, nor does it always fulfill one's expectations. This doesn't mean that a forty- to sixty-year relationship is off to a bad start and is never going to recover. The time of birth is only one moment in the continuing relationship between parents and children, and you still have many days, months, and years ahead of you to love your child.

THREE

Into the Mouths of Babes: Breast Feeding and Bottle Feeding

THERE ARE two ways to feed a baby: at the breast or by bottle. Many women have definite opinions and have made a personal choice even before they become pregnant. Breast feeding is the preferred method today, but there are still women for whom bottle feeding is an appropriate choice. How do these women or others make that decision?

Certainly the most up-to-date medical information should be a factor. Most pediatricians and other health-care professionals recommend breast feeding, and it's the method I recommend to my patients, all other factors being equal. However, there are no absolute rights and wrongs. After reading this chapter, I want you to know that whatever method you choose—even if it is a combination of the two—will be the right one for you.

BREAST FEEDING

There's no doubt that maternal milk is the perfect food. Cow's milk is exactly right for calves, goat's milk is the perfect food for baby goats, and human breast milk is provided by nature for human newborns. It's unheard of for an infant to have trouble digesting human breast milk, and the concentration of protein and minerals is optimal for digestion and metabolic needs.

Breast milk enhances the absorption of important elements needed for growth. When recent studies showed that the iron and zinc content of human milk is quite low, some people thought that breast-fed babies might require supplements of these substances. However, nature's ingenuity was revealed when further studies indicated that a newborn absorbs iron and zinc much more efficiently from breast milk than from a commercial formula.

Breast feeding also enhances the bonding process between mother and child. A more intimate contact is established than with bottle feeding. During the fifteen or twenty minutes it takes for nursing, the baby and mother study each other intently in a profound, loving communication. They are literally skin to skin as physical and emotional nourishment flows between them. There are few other opportunities throughout life for such prolonged close contact. After nourishing her baby *in utero* for nine months, the new mother who breast-feeds feels additional fulfillment in continuing that nourishment. One new mother told me, "My baby gets so agitated and upset when he's hungry. When I put him to the breast and he sucks frantically for a few seconds, then stops and looks at me, it's as if he's saying, 'Thank you.' "

Breast feeding is above all convenient. There are no bottles to wash and store, no nipples to clean. The food is already preheated, the supply virtually endless, and it's easy to carry around. So what are the disadvantages of breast feeding?

A supposed disadvantage is not being able to measure the baby's intake. Actually, however, this is an advantage, because the baby isn't being pressured to finish a predetermined amount of milk. The amount of intake varies from feeding to feeding, and there is no "right amount." Babies are smart; they stop eating when they are full. Your baby is receiving enough calories and fluid if you need to change wet diapers at least six to eight times a day and on your regular office visits your pediatrician assures you that weight gain is adequate.

Although breast milk is a natural product and perfectly designed for babies' needs, we live in an impure world, filled with chemicals and pollutants. Some, like PCB, accumulate in the human body and are excreted through breast milk. If you live in an area where PCB or other contaminants have been detected in the water system or the air, you might want to have your milk tested. Ask your pediatrician for advice about this procedure.

Some people maintain that breast feeding hampers a woman's activities. That's true in a way. But having a baby is what really ties you down! The new mother who breastfeeds is not chained to home; with some creative compromises she should be able to nurse in various environments. After nursing routines are well established, no harm is done if another person gives the baby an occasional bottle of expressed breast milk when it's necessary for mother and baby to be separated.

Another myth is that breast feeding is complicated. A young woman consulted me shortly before the birth of her first baby. As we talked I asked her how she planned to feed her baby. "Well, I was planning to breast feed," she said, "but I had no idea it was so complicated." Surprised, I asked her what she meant by complicated. She answered, "I thought all you needed were breasts and a baby and you put them together. But my friend gave me a book an inch thick to read. And they devoted a whole evening to breast feeding in my childbirth classes. I'm beginning to think it will be easier to bottle-feed."

After reassuring this mother-to-be that her first impression was indeed accurate—she did have all the necessary ingredients for successful nursing—I was struck by how many women must have this attitude. Breast feeding should be as natural and easy and simple as any other bodily function. But it has received so much attention in recent years, it would be easy to think that the process is a complicated. It isn't. Even if you don't make your decision until the moment of birth, your experience will most likely be successful. My best advice is to set aside what you've read and relax and let it happen. If you can do this, you and your baby will find each other delightful companions in a rewarding life experience.

If you know that you want to breast-feed, here are some steps you can take in advance to make the process go more smoothly. Toward the end of your pregnancy you should wear a good support bra in any case, and you might want to begin wearing a nursing bra. This is a firm support bra with a flap that folds down to facilitate nursing. A good support bra that closes in the front does the job just as well, however.

You'll also need a supply of breast pads, easily purchased in your local drug store. When you begin nursing, small amounts of milk will leak from your nipples from time to time. A breast pad inserted in your bra will protect your nipples as well as your clothing.

You can expect your nipples to be tender, even sore, for a week or two. The more elastic and supple your nipples are, the more comfortable your experience will be. In the last month or two of your pregnancy, I suggest massaging your nipples twice a day. Ask your obstetrician to recommend a brand of cream or oil. Safflower oil is good and inexpensive. Avoid creams that contain alcohol, and avoid lanolin if you're sensitive to wool. When you massage, take your nipple between thumb and forefinger, roll it back and forth a bit, and extend the nipple as far as you can. Be firm but gentle. You should not experience any pain. If you do this regularly, your nipples will become more supple.

Exposure to air will cause nipples to firm up and increase their resistance to irritation. At private times, you can simply open the front flap of your nursing bra. Your nipples may be tender in the last weeks of pregnancy anyway, and the presence of air will decrease discomfort.

The size of your breasts doesn't have anything to do with your ability to nurse. Big breasts, small breasts, large nipples, small nipples—all work equally well. Sometimes a woman says, "I don't think I can nurse from both breasts because I have an inverted nipple." Actually, inverted nipples are the exception. What most women call inverted are really just flat nipples—the part of the nipple that should protrude doesn't. If you have flat nipples, here's an exercise you might practice in the month or two before delivery.

Think of your nipple as if it were a clock, and put your thumb and forefinger at three and nine o'clock. Gently but firmly spread your fingers five to ten times, not hard enough to hurt. Then place your fingers at six and twelve o'clock and do the same thing. Repeat this several times a day. Most flat nipples will become somewhat more prominent with this treatment.

Inverted nipples are not merely flat; there's actually a depression where the nipple should be. You can buy breast shields which will gently remodel the surface contour of the nipples if you wear them for one or two months before delivery. Your local La Leche League chapter can provide tips about purchasing these shields. La Leche League is a worldwide organization that encourages breast feeding, and is a valuable resource for information and support for nursing mothers as well as for pediatricians.

Breast Feeding in the Hospital

When you are in the hospital, before delivery is under way, you should tell the nurses whether you want to breast- or bottle-feed. The question of whether a baby should receive water in addition to breast milk arises here. Many members of La Leche League maintain that newborns should ingest only breast milk. I agree that ideally a baby should be breast-fed exclusively in the first weeks of life. However, water in small amounts may be necessary and even healthy for some babies. Those who advocate not giving water to a baby say that the infant may experience "nipple confusion" and refuse the mother's breast. I have not seen this happen. In my experience there has never been any confusion which fluid is tastier and more satisfying. Another argument has it that giving a baby water may interfere with milk production. However, in the first few days after birth, when milk flow may be slow and scanty and nipples sore, a newborn may not take in enough fluid. This can contribute to an elevated jaundice level and possibly a longer hospital stay for treatment of the condition. Not every newborn needs water, but nurses can tell when additional fluid is advisable. Under these circumstances, a judicious amount of water won't interfere with milk production and may prevent minor complications.

After delivery, a mother can nurse as soon as she has fully recovered and is awake. Experiment until you find the position that's comfortable for you. A liberal use of pillows behind your back, on your lap, or next to you may make the first few nursings easier. If you rest repeatedly on one arm, that arm may go to sleep and develop a temporary nerve problem, so it is best to vary your position. If the birth was by cesarean section, you may want to keep a pillow between the baby and your tender tummy.

Babies have a lovely response called the rooting reflex. When an area of the cheek near the mouth is gently stroked, the baby will automatically turn to the side being stroked. If you try to force your baby's mouth toward your breast, the reaction will be to turn the other way. But if you gently stroke the side of your infant's mouth with your nipple, your newborn will turn hungrily to that side, searching for your breast.

Babies know how to suck; in fact they even do it *in utero.* And some babies even start sucking on the obstetrician's finger before they are fully delivered. Even so, babies may need to learn how to suck from the breast. Be sure your baby's mouth contains a good portion of the nipple and not just the central protruding part.

The baby's suckling releases a hormone in the mother's brain which helps the uterus to contract and return to its normal size. The risk of bleeding is reduced. Your uterus, which was the size of a beach ball, must now shrink to the size of a pear. You may experience uterine cramps when your baby first starts to suckle because you are stimulating this process. The suckling also increases the flow of hormones involved with production and release of breast milk.

The first fluid from the breast is called colostrum, a yellowish, watery fluid very high in nutrients. It's particularly high in immunoglobulins which coat the baby's gastrointestinal tract and throat with a mild anti-infective substance and guard against certain bacteria and viruses.

On the first day it might be advisable to limit breast feeding to three to five minutes on each breast. Your nipples may become sore if you nurse longer than that. Over the next three to five days, gradually increase the time to fifteen to twenty minutes per breast.

Nurse alternately from both breasts. Some infants seem to have a definite preference for one breast. Obviously there is no difference in the milk. The explanation could be that the milk flows more readily from one side than from the other, or that the shape of one nipple may be slightly different.

How often should you nurse your baby? Whenever he or she is hungry. In the hospital where I do most of my work, babies room in with their mothers, which means they are with their mothers, except when the mothers are showering, sleeping, or otherwise indisposed. When mother and baby are together, the baby's own schedule is the criterion for when to feed. Some hospitals, however, will keep newborns in the nursery for two or three hours at a time and bring them out for feedings, putting the infants on the hospital's schedule and not their own. This unfortunate practice is diminishing, and most hospitals routinely allow babies to room in with their mothers.

Breasts are somewhat firm the first few days after delivery. Then, after a period ranging from two days to a week, they may become engorged. Engorged breasts feel (and are) extremely full, may leak, and feel as though they must be emptied because the milk has "come in."

When the baby sucks, a response called a "let-down reflex" occurs. The baby's nursing, or sometimes even the baby's crying, stimulates a brain hormone that releases milk from the breast. You will feel more relaxed when this process begins and your breasts are relieved of the urgent need to be emptied. Now the baby is receiving classical breast milk instead of merely colostrum.

After a week you can expect to be feeding your baby about ten to twenty minutes on each breast, or a total of twenty to forty minutes per feeding. Mothers often ask me how they can adjust their newborn to a nursing schedule. I tell them that the baby already has a schedule—its own. Babies are not gas tanks that are filled up, run three hours, and then need refueling. Two infants of the same age may nurse at different intervals, one every hour and the other every three hours. Or a baby whose schedule was every three hours for weeks may suddenly be hungry every hour.

Breast feeding is a supply-and-demand system. The more the baby demands, the more milk will be produced. If an infant wants to nurse every hour, some women worry that their milk is inadequate and supplement with formula. Formula remains in the stomach longer than breast milk, which is digested much more quickly. Some mothers then continue to supplement with formula because, they say, "my breast milk must be inadequate. Look how contented my baby is with formula—he's sleeping for three hours."

However, if you interrupt this natural supply-and-demand cycle, you will lessen your milk production, which will then indeed be inadequate. Let your baby set the schedule. If you find that nursing every hour exhausts you, consult your pediatrician or La Leche League before adding formula feedings.

After the baby has nursed from one breast, allow the baby to burp. This releases air taken in from sucking. Then let the baby nurse from the other breast. Some infants will give you a terrific burp as soon as you hold them upright. Others will take fifteen minutes for results. That's about the time limit for burping—if you haven't gotten a burp in fifteen minutes, forget about it. Every baby doesn't have to burp at every feeding.

Breast Feeding at Home

Life with a newborn is sure to be hectic and unsettled. When nursing mothers say they have problems, I ask them how many people are coming to visit the baby or how much attention they're giving to household matters. I invariably discover that these mothers are trying to do too much. This is a fact of life for new parents. Nearly all are sleep-deprived, have disrupted households, and feel far from serene.

A relaxed environment is very important for both mother and child because stress can affect breast-milk production. Relaxation promotes production of milk, and tension retards it. Since your primary task is to nurse your baby, ask others to help with housework and routine daily chores. If grandparents are visiting, they might take care of the grocery shopping or the laundry. One thing you must accept: now that you have a baby, you will *never* again get everything done. Patients sometimes ask if they should hire a nurse for the weeks after delivery. What they really need is a housekeeper. It's much more important for you to concentrate on your baby's needs rather than on the dusting. If you wear a robe at home (and why not settle on a pretty one), you'll convey the message that you're not functioning as a homemaker but as a new mother who is recovering and relaxing.

When you breast-feed, find a spot in the home where you're most comfortable. That might be the lounger in the den, a rocking chair in the baby's room, or on your bed. In the first few weeks, while you're adjusting to nursing, you should have relative privacy and be either by yourself or with only the father. Give yourself plenty of time; don't try to rush. It may take fifteen or twenty minutes for you and your newborn just to settle down and start nursing. Your baby may fall asleep after a minute or two and may need to be awakened to finish the feeding. While you nurse, try to forget everything else.

We can use the word *relax* all we want, but how do we do it on demand? There are physical ways to unwind: take a warm shower, or sit in a warm tub; walk around the block, or go for a swim. Whatever feels good to you and makes you feel as though you're doing something just for yourself is right. Some women claim that drinking beer is good for milk production. It seems to be true but not because there's anything special about beer. The extra fluid and the mild dose of alcohol may relax you a bit, which will help your milk to flow. A small glass of wine or beer in the evening may help you to unwind, and it won't harm your baby. But don't overdo it with alcohol.

Many new fathers feel left out when their partners are breast-feeding. Before the baby arrived, the father was the primary love object. Now this little bundle is monopolizing all the mother's time and attention. Even though the father's feelings may have no rational basis, it's not unusual for men to feel rejected, perhaps even jealous. Mothers and fathers both need to remember to care for each other while they're caring for their baby.

This is a time when the father's presence is of special significance. New mothers often feel frightened, inadequate, and unsure about their roles and responsibilities. Couples need to listen to each other's anxieties, reassure each other of their competence, and look forward to being wonderful parents, learning along the way together.

Some women ask about the effect breast feeding will have on sexual desire. The truth is that most women don't feel very sexy in the first few weeks after delivery, whether they're breast-feeding or not. And, once you have a baby, your sex life is forever changed. Spontaneity goes out the window, energy is frequently diverted, and interruptions are frequent. Yet your feelings of fulfillment as a woman, both sexual and social, can be so augmented by successful nursing that breast feeding may actually have a positive influence so far as closeness to your partner is concerned.

Mothers who breast-feed should drink plenty of fluids, but diet doesn't really have to be altered. After the first few days, your natural thirst mechanism will take over, and you may feel a great thirst while you're nursing. In fact, many women place a glass of water nearby before they nurse because they know they'll get thirsty during the feeding.

New mothers have to consume about 500 extra calories per day while they're nursing, and ideally your diet should be high in complex carbohydrates, low in fat, high in calcium, and a little higher in protein than if you weren't nursing. However, there's nothing you can't eat while you're breast-feeding. Simply use your common sense. For example, if you notice that your baby cries all night whenever you eat garlic, don't eat garlic. You should cut down on coffee and caffeine-containing colas, otherwise your baby may be wakeful and fretful. When patients ask me, "Can I eat chocolate?" I always say that life without chocolate isn't worth living. Breast-fed babies in many different cultures appear to thrive on breast milk, whether their mothers eat spicy Thai saté or fried plantain.

Let your hunger mechanism plus the scales dictate how much you eat. Beyond the initial weight loss right after delivery, it's difficult to lose weight when you're nursing. Unless you have a significant health problem such as high blood pressure that requires you to lose weight, put off reducing until after you've weaned your baby.

Certain medications should be avoided while you're nursing because they are secreted through breast milk. Check with your pediatrician to find out if any prescription drug you are taking is safe for your infant. Elements we'd like babies to get, such as fluoride, don't pass readily into breast milk. Unfortunately, harmful substances, like nicotine and drugs, do.

Women often think that there is no need for birth control while they are nursing. This isn't true. While most women don't have periods while they nurse, a woman is still fertile and can become pregnant. Your obstetrician can advise you as to which is the best method of birth control while nursing.

Avoid smoking while you're breast-feeding. Nicotine and its breakdown products are transferred to the baby in breast milk. In fact, this might be a good time to quit smoking forever.

A few minor problems may accompany breast feeding. You may have a sore, hard spot on your breast if one of the milk ducts has become plugged. Warm compresses will relieve the discomfort. If the area becomes red or feels warm, or if you run a fever, the clogged duct may be infected. In that case, your doctor will usually prescribe an antibiotic and hot packs. Nursing helps to relieve clogged ducts, so continue to nurse as usual from that breast unless you find that the milk takes on a brownish color.

A crack or small ulcer may develop on the nipple, which can be extremely uncomfortable. If it's too painful for you to nurse from the sore breast, you can use a nipple shield, which looks like a bottle nipple. When placed over your own nipple, it produces an airtight seal. The baby's sucking can draw out your milk without contact with your own nipple. However, these shields may not work well and may even cause more discomfort. In that case, for a day or two express milk by hand from that breast until the nipple heals. If your nipples are sore, be sure to keep them dry. Change the breast pad inside your bra frequently. Expose your nipples to the air when you can, and use a lubricating cream to keep the tissues soft.

Clothing When Nursing

Unless you own your own dry-cleaning establishment, the clothes you wear while you're nursing should be washable. Not only will breast milk stain your blouse, but your baby will invariably and unpredictably spit up on you at the most inopportune times. Recently, a patient with a one-month-old baby was in my office for the first time. After introducing ourselves, I said, "This is your first baby, I see."

"How did you know?" she asked.

I replied, "Because you're wearing a beautiful white wool suit."

The clothing you wear should be easily adjusted. There are cleverly designed tops that have concealed slits through which you can nurse discreetly. These are available at maternity and children's shops. However, any front-closing top or dress or a sweater that lifts easily from the bottom is quite satisfactory.

Loose tops that aren't revealing or form-fitting will be the most comfortable and look the best. While you're nursing, your breasts will change size every few hours.

Breast Feeding in Public

In a medical magazine there was a story about a little boy who watched while his mother was dressing and pointed to her breasts. He said, "I know why you have those. You used them to feed me and my brother." Then he added, "There's something I don't understand. Why did you keep them?"

If everyone remembered what breasts are really there for, there might not be such a fuss about women nursing in public. Since bottle feeding has predominated until recently, we have become unused to breast feeding in public, and some people are offended by it. But we can help if we demonstrate sensitivity to other people's feelings by breast feeding in public areas that offer the most privacy. For example, if you're dining out with a nursing baby, try to sit at a table or booth far away from the busiest area, facing away from the center of the room.

Breast Feeding at Work

Nursing in public may also involve nursing on the job, if you're fortunate enough to have the kind of job where your baby can be with you. One of my patients is the registrar of a liberal college of the arts. Her baby was with her in her office all day, and nursed on demand. This woman's breast feeding was one of the least radical activities at that school and fit in with the college's progressive philosophy. Naturally, not everyone works for such an open-minded employer.

Depending on your work atmosphere, you have three possible choices.

The first option is to stop nursing when you return to work. Of course, it's best to wean your baby gradually. After all, you don't want the baby to lose your company and your breast at the same time. After two or three months of nursing at home, plan on a month to wean your baby before your return to work. Stop the daytime feedings first, but continue the morning and evening nursings until the end of the weaning period. This will be most comfortable for you.

The second option is to nurse your baby while you're home and have the baby bottle-fed while you're on the job. This way the baby still receives some breast milk, you can still have the fulfillment and pleasure of coming home and nursing, and separation between mother and infant is more gradual. About two weeks before returning to work, stop the breast feedings during those hours when you will be at work. If your breasts are uncomfortable during weaning at home, you can manually express enough milk occasionally to maintain comfort. Within one to three weeks, you'll find that your milk supply will adapt to the demands of your baby. You'll have sufficient milk when you're home without experiencing leaking from engorged breasts during work hours.

The third option, to express breast milk while you're on the job, requires some dedication on your part and cooperation from your employer. It may be worth it if you have the required privacy and facilities for storage. You'll need to spend twenty to thirty minutes twice a day pumping your breasts. In a fairly small workplace, especially one that is managed by women, you may be able to arrange this. I've had a variety of patients who have combined work and breast feeding. They include teachers, lawyers, doctors, and telephone-company employees.

How do you express your milk? The natural way is to express milk manually into a small glass or baby's bottle by rhythmic squeezing of your breast and nipple. This method —not the most efficient one—doesn't use any suction, takes a long time, and often produces very little milk.

You can use a manual breast pump. One type resembles a bicycle horn, is made of plastic and has a rubber bulb on the end. When you squeeze and release the bulb, suction is created. But this kind of pump doesn't work very well since you can't easily control the degree of suction. The second kind is more expensive but works better. It's about the size of a baby's bottle, is made of plastic, and looks like a bicycle pump. It's flared to fit over your nipple, and requires two hands to use: one hand holds the phlanged end tightly against the nipple while the other produces the suction and pumping action to withdraw the milk. This pump, usually very effective, can be bought for about $20 at your local pharmacy. There are several brands: Happy Family and Care-All are two.

An electric breast pump is the most effective alternative. Since large pumps cost between $800 and $1,000, most people rent the mechanism for about $2 a day plus an additional $10 or so for the reusable receptacles. You can rent them from pharmacies or a local La Leche League chapter. A small pump, such as Gerber's "Precious Care," can be purchased for about $40.00.

It takes about ten to fifteen minutes to empty a breast with an electric pump, and it only requires one hand. It works essentially the same as a manual pump but more efficiently. A piston goes back and forth, producing a gentle, rhythmic suction, which extracts the milk from your breast just as a baby would.

Plan to start pumping your breasts a week before you return to work so that you'll have a supply of milk on hand. Nurse your baby from one breast, and pump the other at each feeding. Breast milk, once expressed, should not be stored longer than a week in a self-defrosting freezer but can be stored indefinitely in a deep freeze.

Once the milk has thawed, whatever is not used should be discarded. Storage containers must be scrupulously clean; they don't have to be sterilized, but must be scrubbed and dishwasher clean. Disposable plastic containers such as Playtex Baby Nursers are best, are easily frozen and defrosted, and are ready to use (no changing of containers). Breast milk expressed at work for use at home should be transported frozen in an insulated ice chest.

When to Stop Nursing

Ultimately you have to decide how long to breast-feed. There's no time limit. This will depend on what seems best for you and your child. Most women nurse from six to twelve months. In my opinion, it would be the best of all possible worlds if you could breast-feed for at least nine to twelve months until it is time for the baby to drink from a cup.

Some mothers will differ with this recommendation, especially committed members of La Leche League. If you ask these women how long they nurse their children, many will say, "Until the age of three." Clearly, nursing at these later ages is not primarily nutritional but largely psychological—mother is acting as a kind of fast-food stand and comfort station for the child. The process of nursing involves a complex interaction of mother's and infant's needs. Breast feeding becomes just as important to some women as it is to their babies.

Women who are still nursing after eighteen months or so might do well to examine their motivations. Are they doing this because the child demands it, or are they reluctant to have their child grow up? The process of growing up involves small gradual separations. If you hold on too tightly, you won't allow your son or daughter the room to grow. If your child is upset and feels the need to nurse—and you're comfortable with it—by all means don't deny the need. But if you're offering your breast to a toddler who is basically disinterested or you're breast-feeding out of laziness, habit, or for some psychological need of your own, you may not be doing what's best in the long run for either your baby or yourself.

A few years ago a three-year-old who had not been breast-fed for a year came to see me. She was told she would receive a shot and stoically accepted the news with barely a whimper. But then she turned to her mother with tear-filled eyes and said, "Mom, I need to nurse." She climbed up on her mother's lap, nursed for a few seconds, then jumped off and was ready for the shot.

Some children wean themselves—they no longer want the breast at nine months or a year or fifteen months. This is often difficult for mothers, who can feel a sense of rejection. The length of time for nursing depends on what is satisfactory for both mother and baby.

Women who nurse beyond six or nine months tell me they are frequently besieged by other women who ask, "Oh, are you still breast-feeding?"

On the other hand, another patient told me of the opposite kind of interference. The baby's grandmother said, "I hope you nurse *our* baby for at least a year."

The pressure that other people bring to bear on nursing women may stem from their own feelings of inadequacy as parents. A woman who hasn't nursed her infant may need to reassure herself that she isn't less of a mother. When people ask if you're still nursing, all you need to do is smile, nod, and say, "Yes, and my baby and I are both enjoying it very much." Don't let others influence you on such an intimate matter!

You chose to nurse because it feels right for you. You continue to breast-feed because you and your child enjoy it and because your feelings of fulfillment, closeness to your child, and adequacy as a mother are gratified. The time to stop is when you and your child mutually agree that these needs have been met.

BOTTLE FEEDING

Breast feeding may be the preferred method of infant feeding, but it certainly isn't mandatory. A woman may choose to bottle-feed for a number of reasons: personal preference, what fits best with her way of life, or a desire to give the father more time with his newborn. Some women think that bottle feeding means greater freedom, but, as I've said earlier, this isn't necessarily the case. However, in situations such as these, feelings are often more important than fact.

Occasionally a woman has no choice. She cannot breast-feed and has to bottle-feed. If you're taking a medication that might be harmful to the baby, such as an antithyroid drug for an overactive thyroid, you will have to rely on formula. If the prospect of breast feeding makes you anxious, it may not work for you. The good news is that formula is there for you and your baby.

Bottle feeding, when undertaken properly, can provide the same psychological benefits as breast feeding. If you cuddle your baby and talk and look into his or her eyes during the feeding, your baby will feel secure, loved, and satisfied emotionally as well as physically.

There is one clear disadvantage to bottle feeding: it is more expensive than breast feeding. So if cost is a matter of concern for you, this would be a factor to consider when making your decision.

Preparation for Bottle Feeding

You'll need to have a supply of bottles and nipples on hand, and you'll need to know how to prepare formula. Glass bottles are easiest to clean thoroughly, but they can break. Plastic bottles are safer. The cleanest, easiest, and safest plastic containers are the disposable ones like Playtex Baby Nursers or Evenflo Disposable Bottles since you use the little bags once and discard them. Most women I see in my practice use plastic bottles or nursers.

Infants can show a definite preference for certain kinds of nipples. The traditional nipple may be too long for some babies' mouths and cause them to gag. The shorter nipples, such as those manufactured under the brand name Nuk, are touted as orthodontically designed but are really no better unless your baby responds positively to them. The ones on nurser bottles may be more comfortable. Experiment with one or two kinds to find the one that works best for your "nipple gourmet."

Any of the major commercial formulas, such as Enfamil, Similac, and SMA, is fine. Each in its own way comes close to human milk. Unprocessed cow's milk is inappropriate for babies—it is too concentrated and contains a protein molecule that is hard for newborns and babies under six months to digest. In commercial formula, cow's milk is broken down into smaller, more digestible parts. If a history of allergy to cow's milk runs in your family, it may be wise to choose a formula that is made of soy protein. Consult your pediatrician about this.

Commercial formulas come in three forms: powder, concentrate, and ready-to-feed.

I recommend powdered formula because it is the cheapest and easiest to use. Powdered formula is easy to transport, and there are no hidden costs due to the addition of water. You need only mix one bottle at a time, and you can use lukewarm water straight from the tap. Powdered formula doesn't spoil as quickly as formula from an open can. Whether you use tap or bottled water depends on the nature of your water supply. Well water sometimes contains too many minerals for babies' health, and certain municipal waters would be better if charcoal-filtered. Your pediatrician can assess the quality of the water in your community.

If you choose formula in concentrate, be sure to read the container label carefully and add the correct amount of water. If you don't add enough, the formula will be too concentrated for your baby; if you add too much, the mixture won't be sufficiently nourishing. Once you open a can of concentrate, you must mix up several bottles, store them in the refrigerator, and use them within twenty-four hours.

Ready-to-feed is the most convenient formula because it is ready to go with no additions. It is also the most expensive. After you open a can, you must use it all within the time stated on the label. Always, always, always read and reread the instructions on whatever container you're using. Check the expiration date, and don't assume that because you thought you bought ready-to-feed in the store, that's the kind you actually brought home. Make sure the label coincides with what you think you have. I get calls all the time from mothers who have just finished a feeding, only to discover that they had used straight concentrate instead of ready-to-feed or that the formula had expired. Nothing adverse has happened so far, but you can avoid unnecessary worry if you read the label *every* time.

Some mothers still mix their own formula from evaporated milk, sugar, and water. This is just as nutritious as commercial formula, but preparation is so time-consuming and cumbersome that the saving in cost is probably not worth it. Besides, as one of my patients discovered, the evaporated milk never comes out even. This woman's family was eating an awful lot of pudding to use up the extra evaporated milk.

Formula Feeding in the Hospital

In the hospital, your baby's first feeding is usually water. We do this because in rare cases babies may have a problem with the esophagus or stomach that causes them to spit up or choke. There is less cause for concern if the first feeding is only water. Subsequent hospital feedings will be the "house formula" (as in "house wine" or "house dressing"). There is no reason to think that a house formula is better because a hospital is using it. Generally the hospital adopts a brand because that particular formula company landed a contract with that particular hospital.

At first, babies ingest anywhere from half an ounce of formula to an ounce and a half at a feeding. It is almost unheard of for a newborn to finish a four-ounce bottle. If your baby spits up the formula, a different kind may be prescribed. Some infants demonstrate a sensitivity to processed cow's-milk formula as early as the first day.

Formula-fed babies go longer between feedings than breast-fed babies—two to four hours may elapse before they are hungry again, while breast-fed babies may be hungry every hour. Whatever the interval, when the baby is hungry, the baby should be fed. Infants who are rooming in with their mothers can be fed on demand, rather than waiting for the nurse to bring them from the nursery. I, therefore, encourage mothers in the hospital to be with their babies as much as possible.

Bottle Feeding at Home

There is one nice feature of bottle feeding at home: someone else can take over for you when you need help. In contrast to breast feeding, you aren't awakened every time the baby is hungry, and you'll have more chance to recharge your energy than the nursing mother.

In the first several weeks, bottle-fed babies take one to three ounces per feeding every three to four hours. The amount and frequency may vary from feeding to feeding. Smaller babies need smaller, more frequent feedings than larger newborns. When parents ask me how to set up a bottle-feeding schedule, I tell them, as I do parents of breast-feeding babies, that the baby is already on a schedule—its own. An infant will let you know when it's time to eat. Although formula may remain longer in a baby's stomach than breast milk, that doesn't mean that two ounces of formula will last two hours and four ounces will last four hours.

If you are a lucky parent and your newborn sleeps through the night right from the beginning, by all means enjoy your good fortune and don't wake the baby for a feeding. You might also refrain from bragging about this to your friends who aren't so lucky. However, your baby shouldn't sleep for long periods during the day. After four hours, if the infant does not spontaneously awaken for feeding, you might change diapers, remove warm clothing, or use a cool washcloth on the baby's face and head. This will stimulate the baby to awaken without feeling disturbed and will give you a better chance for a longer sleep at night.

With commercial formula, sterilization of equipment and utensils is not necessary as long as they are kept scrupulously clean. Many people still believe in sterilization, and I am embarrassed when I find I haven't told them otherwise. Often, at a four-month checkup, mothers will ask if they can stop sterilizing now. I haven't the heart to tell them it wasn't necessary in the first place, so I give them permission to stop. If you use plastic or glass bottles, scrub them well with a brush and soap in hot water, and rinse them thoroughly or wash them in an automatic dishwasher. If you have a good dishwasher, automatic or human, and the nipples are washed and rinsed thoroughly, they will be clean enough.

Some dishwashers are equipped with a special small cage just for nipples. If yours doesn't have this, you can use a lingerie bag, well secured in the dishwasher. Fill nipples with water, and give them a squeeze to make sure that water squirts through and milk isn't clogging the hole. If a whitish residue accumulates on your bottles, soak them for a few hours in a solution of vinegar and water.

Commercial formula doesn't need to be heated, and some babies even seem to like cold milk. But if the baby prefers it warm, it need be no warmer than 80 degrees Fahrenheit. The safest way to heat a bottle is to put a pan of water on the stove or in the microwave and then place the bottle in the pan of hot water for a few minutes. If you warm the bottle itself in the microwave, be very careful; leave the top off and carefully test the temperature on the inside of your wrist or with the tip of your tongue. Microwave ovens heat liquids very quickly, turning the water to steam, and the contents can explode when the bottle is removed from the oven. Even without such a dramatic result, the formula may still be too hot for the baby's mouth and esophagus. My advice is *always* to test it!

The Family's Role in Bottle Feeding

Bottle feeding can enhance a father's bonding with his newborn and increase his sense of competence and participation. Many men feel uncertain about holding a small infant. Some new fathers initially handle their babies as if they were holding a Ming vase and wearing boxing gloves. But once a father gives his baby a bottle and the baby relaxes and stares gratefully into his eyes, his feelings of clumsiness quickly evaporate.

Some Fine Points of Bottle Feeding

It is possible to overfeed a bottle baby, especially if parents feel that each bottle has to be emptied. Remember that every whimper doesn't necessarily mean hunger. Babies who are overfed will have stomach pains, may vomit, or may gain too much weight. If you overfeed, the more that is ingested, the more uncomfortable the baby becomes, and a vicious cycle begins. To avoid this, remove the bottle when the infant seems to be finished, even if some formula remains. When the baby fusses for attention shortly after a feeding, investigate other possibilities. The baby may want to be held or to suck on a pacifier or to be changed.

Don't try to rush through a feeding; it's a precious time. Never ever prop up a bottle near the baby and walk away. This practice is dangerous—the infant can choke, and (equally important) you have lost an opportunity for the warmth and closeness that are so emotionally significant to your developing relationship. Hold your baby in your arms during feedings. If a baby drinks while he or she is lying flat, ear infections can develop if milk flows to the back of the throat and irritates the opening to the middle ear.

Tip the bottle so that the nipple is completely filled with formula. If air and milk mix in the nipple, the baby will swallow excess air and may have gas pains or excessive belching or may spit up.

Bottle-fed babies should be burped about halfway through the bottle and again when the bottle is finished. Some babies are great burpers, and others will take what seems like all day for one measly little burp.

How and When to Wean

Weaning refers to the transition period from breast to bottle to cup. From about nine months to a year, most children should be able to use a training cup, a covered plastic cup with a spout. If you try to introduce a normal cup, the contents will probably end up on the floor because a baby's motor coordination is not sufficiently developed for the use of a regular cup. After nine months is a good time to start the training cup, when several teeth have come in. This time is right because bottle feeding is not the best thing for a baby's new teeth. Toddlers who are still sucking on a bottle all day or snacking during the night can develop a condition called "nursing-bottle mouth." A constant stream of milk or juice in the baby's mouth causes erosion of the tooth enamel, creating premature cavities and severe enamel destruction. If your toddler demands a bottle before going to bed, let the child have a bottle, finish it, and them remove it from the crib. Once we thought nursing-bottle mouth only occurred with formula-fed babies, but recently the same syndrome was observed in a breast-fed sixteen month old who slept with her mother. Whenever the toddler was hungry, she reached for her mother's breast and developed the same kind of dental problems seen in bottle-fed babies with nursing-bottle mouth.

If your child initially rejects the training cup, don't try to force the issue. Reintroduce the cup gently and positively at weekly intervals until the child accepts it. You can ease the transition by gradually decreasing the amount of milk in the bottle and increasing the amount in the cup. Between the ages of one and two, most children adapt and slowly but surely give up the bottle. The length of time for weaning will depend on how many bottles a day babies drink and how attached they are to their bottles. Some children like to drink small amounts frequently and a child who is attached to a bottle all through the day will take longer to wean than one who only drinks at scheduled mealtimes. The most treasured bottles are usually the ones just before the baby goes to sleep. Since these are related to relaxation as well as nourishment, the bedtime and naptime bottles are usually the last to go. Just keep in mind that weaning should be gradual—a slow transition—and if you're patient, loving, and encouraging, you will make it easier for your child to take this next step toward independence.

FOUR

Mealtime and the First Year: How to Avoid Peas in Your Hair

BIRTH TO SIX MONTHS

BREAST MILK or formula are all that babies need for the first six months. After that, they initially need foods that are high in iron, so we start solid feedings with iron-fortified rice cereal such as Gerber or Beech-Nut. Between four and six months, start with a tablespoon of dry rice cereal mixed with either breast milk, formula, or apple juice, and feed this to the baby once a day. Continue the usual breast or bottle feedings, and after several weeks increase the cereal mixture to twice a day.

Breakfast, with its atmosphere of preparation for the day,

probably isn't the best time to introduce solid foods, because spoon feedings take longer than breast or bottle feeding. Lunchtime or midafternoon, when your household is less hectic, may be a more convenient time. Use a small spoon, and give the baby time to get used to the unfamiliar cereal taste. In relaxed surroundings your baby will learn that mealtimes are fun, occasions for enjoying each other's company and sharing new experiences.

If you taste the cereal yourself, you'll find that it's barely palatable. But don't let your own adult tastes be the guide for what should appeal to your infant. Because cereal is so bland, some people mix it with bananas or some other sweet fruit. But I don't think that's a good idea. It teaches your child to expect bland foods to be sweetened. Babies willingly accept bland food, and we should encourage that trait for as long as possible.

Rice cereal can be constipating, in which case you can try barley or oatmeal instead. Once or twice a day for cereal is enough until after six months.

SIX TO NINE MONTHS

Now you can increase the amount and variety of puréed food. I recommend starting with vegetables instead of fruits; your baby is more likely to accept bland vegetables if you introduce the sweeter fruits later as a dessert. It doesn't matter in what order you introduce vegetables; spinach, squash, green beans, carrots are all about the same. You will soon learn that no matter what you do, your child has definite preferences. Some infants love peas and spit out green beans, and others will devour green beans and spit peas in your face.

A long-time, beloved patient of mine has four children, each with distinctive attitudes toward food. One child, a finicky eater who would accept only a few foods, was so persnickety that he fussed about how they were served and what utensils were used. Her last child, on the other hand, ate everything in sight and wasn't above stealing food from the other children's plates.

Introduce new foods slowly, at the rate of one every three to five days. Some foods may not sit right with your child or may even cause an allergic reaction, and you'll be better able to figure out which food caused the problem if new items are introduced gradually and separately. Start with a tablespoon full of peas, for example. If the child enjoys them, serve the baby a quarter to a half a jar once or twice a day for the next two or three days. You can use commercial jarred food or make it yourself, which we'll discuss later. After you've offered a number of different vegetables, turn to fruits: mash a ripe banana or a very soft pear, or use jarred commercial peaches or pears. During this period your baby should be eating solids twice a day, perhaps with cereal and fruit for the first meal and vegetables and fruit for the second. There's no prescribed order, but citrus fruits, such as oranges, lemons, and grapefruit, have a tendency to give infants rashes and allergic reactions. Avoid them until your child is at least one year old.

As solid-food intake increases, the frequency of breast or bottle feeding will decrease, but your child will still need about eighteen to twenty-four ounces of formula or milk each day. By nine months to a year, if about one-third of your baby's diet is in the form of solid food, cow's milk can be substituted for breast milk or formula.

Should babies start on whole, low-fat, or nonfat milk? The medical literature gives conflicting advice, but I favor low-fat milk. The general American diet is high in cholesterol and other saturated animal fats, which contribute to later vascular disease such as hypertension and heart trouble. Low-fat milk removes some of the animal fat from cow's milk but not too much; nonfat milk is virtually without fat. Children do need a certain amount of fat, and a diet that's too restrictive may impair growth and development. Whole milk contains a considerable amount of animal fat. So, in my view, it's healthiest to lower cholesterol intake from the very beginning by drinking low-fat milk.

Raw (unpasteurized) milk is an absolute no-no. The purported benefits of raw milk are dubious, and the risk of a disease from raw milk is very *real.* Advocates of raw milk argue that the cows are inspected regularly, which does minimize the possibility of some bacteria being transmitted. But other organisms, especially salmonella, a bacteria that causes bone and intestinal infections, grow easily in unsterile dairy products, and most outbreaks of salmonella these days can be traced to raw milk.

Yogurt, on the other hand, is a marvelous snack food for infants and toddlers. Yogurt, by itself or mixed with fresh or puréed fruit, is better than the kind with fruit and sugar already added.

NINE TO TWELVE MONTHS

You can introduce egg yolk now. Avoid egg whites until a child is more than a year old. The whites often produce allergic reactions in younger children. Limit egg yolks to two or three times a week because of their high fat content.

In the nine-to-twelve-month period meats come next. White meat, especially turkey, chicken, and veal, is unlikely to cause an allergic reaction and should be introduced first. Use jarred commercial baby food, or put some white meat through a hand grinder so the baby can share the family's chicken dinner. I always have a large Thanksgiving dinner crowd, and my friends with infants bring their hand grinder so their babies can enjoy the turkey with us. Beef, lamb, and other red meats can be introduced later. These are stronger in taste, so babies may not like them as much at first, and they have more fat. Red meats, however, are the best source of iron in the diet, so three servings a week is a reasonable amount. Babies don't have to eat meat every day, and some babies don't like meat at all. I assure parents of these babies that vegetarians are generally healthy, and as long as babies are being fed some animal protein in milk and eggs, their diet is quite adequate.

Beans, such as kidney or pinto beans, and lentils, cooked until soft, are good sources of protein and can be used as substitutes for meat. Cooked lentils are easily puréed in a blender or food processor, and soft beans can be mashed with a fork.

Around nine months, babies use two fingers to pick up small objects and put them in their mouths, whether the objects are edible or not. To capitalize on this, we introduce small pieces of soft "finger foods": the ever-popular Cheerios, soft pieces of very ripe pear, small pieces of well-cooked carrot, slices of bananas or other soft fruit with the skin removed.

There are certain finger foods your toddler should not eat until at least age three because they can get caught in a small child's throat. The major culprits are nuts, popcorn, firm pieces of carrot, corn or other hard vegetables, raisins, round pieces of hot dog or pieces of meat larger than one-quarter inch, and whole grapes.

At nine months some babies like lumpier, chunky foods, such as cottage cheese, finely ground hamburger mixed with mashed potato, and soft carrots mashed with a fork.

You can use commercial "junior foods" or prepare the food yourself.

ONE YEAR

By this time your toddler should be eating three meals a day along with the family. Small amounts of several foods at each meal will provide variety and a good nutritional balance. You can bring out the egg white and citrus now, and introduce fish without bones, poached, steamed, or broiled. The type of food a toddler eats now depends largely on physical development. Molars don't come in until a child is close to two, so steak or roast beef or lettuce will be a problem. But toddlers can chew ground meat or cooked chicken or turkey cut in small pieces. Other possibilities are toast and soft cheese—the old reliable grilled-cheese sandwich—and soft vegetables. Baked or boiled potatoes without butter, salt, or sour cream are a good source of iron and fiber and almost always popular with the one-year-old crowd.

Between-meal snacks should be the same food you would serve at a meal. Instead of cookies, candies, and sweets, offer small pieces of cheese, fruit, yogurt, or soft vegetables.

FOODS TO AVOID

Babies under one year should not be fed honey. Whether filtered or unfiltered, organic or not, honey contains botulism spores. Only in infants—not in older children—these spores release a toxin that causes infant botulism, a serious illness.

Peanut butter has a tendency to stick in the back of the mouth and may cause a child under two to gag and choke.

Don't start a dessert habit. If you want to end a meal with

something special, serve a piece of fruit instead of puddings or custards. As we know, most desserts are high in fats and calories and low in essential nutrition. If you encourage a sweet tooth in infancy, the resulting eating habits are hard to break later.

Processed meats such as sausages and luncheon meats are high in salt. So are canned and frozen foods. Although some frozen foods may not have added salt, the process of freezing raises the salt content, sometimes as much as ten times. If you use commercial baby foods in jars, be sure to buy brands with "No salt or sugar added" displayed on the label.

Some people believe that health-food-store food is better than that from a supermarket. Fresh fruits and vegetables from the supermarket are just as good and less expensive than so-called health foods. If you want to give your baby the best, avoid frozen, canned, and processed foods, and buy lovely fresh fruits and vegetables.

SAFETY MEASURES

If you use commercial baby foods, don't feed your child directly from the jar. Enzymes and bacteria from the baby's mouth will be introduced into the jar. Enzymes make the food watery, and bacteria cause the food to spoil more quickly. Put a few spoonfuls on a plate, and feed the baby from the dish. After the feeding, refrigerate the opened jar and discard what's left on the plate.

Dried baby food is now being introduced to supermarkets. You can remove enough for just one feeding and mix it with water to any desired consistency. If these become popular, it may solve the problem of spoilage.

Children should never be left alone when they're eating,

nor should they be allowed—once they're ambulatory—to walk around carrying food. Children choke easily, and an adult should always be right there to help.

HOW TO MAKE YOUR OWN BABY FOOD

To purée vegetables, steam them in a small amount of water without added salt or butter. Drain the vegetables, and save the liquid. Purée the vegetables in the blender, and add a little of the reserved liquid for smoothness and to restore some of the nutrients lost in cooking.

When you purée several servings at once, which is usually the case in a blender or food processor, freeze the extra portions in an ice-cube tray. Frozen, the cubes can be stored in a plastic bag in your freezer and thawed one or two cubes at a time.

You can freeze almost any vegetable this way, but not fruits. A few fruits like apples or prunes must be cooked before they can be puréed, but most other's don't need puréeing if they're ripe. Fresh fruit like bananas, papaya, or peaches can be mashed with a fork or ground in a food mill, after the skin is removed. Puréed fruit doesn't freeze well, so it's best to make only one serving at a time.

Sometimes your baby can share the chicken or turkey or ground meat, potatoes or rice, and cooked vegetables from the family table. Many foods can be easily ground in a food mill or baby-food grinder available at a baby supply store. Most red meat, however, doesn't grind easily this way; you may have to rely on commercial jarred red meats.

When I was a resident, the Scandinavian mother of a six month old asked if she could make her own food, to which I, of course, said, "Yes." A few months later, I asked her what her baby was eating.

"Puréed filet, asparagus, whatever my husband and I eat," she said. Lucky baby. But babies don't need to be such gourmets and will be healthy and content with simple fruits, vegetables, and modest portions of meat.

INDIVIDUAL VARIATIONS IN APPETITE

When children have more mobility, there will be times when they seem to be eating absolutely nothing. Some parents are convinced they will soon have a starving waif, yet these children of reduced appetite, with their lovely little tree-stump legs and sausage fingers, are obviously not wasting away.

Children do go through periods when you can count their daily caloric intake on one hand. There are several reasons for this. In the first year, babies double their birth weight by the age of six months and triple it by a year. For example, a baby who weighed eight pounds at birth will be sixteen pounds at six months and twenty-four pounds at one year. That's an extraordinary increase—300 percent in a year. Growth rate then slows down, which is a good thing or you'd have a monster two year old. This slowdown in growth is accompanied by a slowdown in eating.

Also, at the ages of one to three, most toddlers are whirlwinds of activity, in motion from sunup to sundown. Suppose you as an adult were invited to sit down to a meal of steak and potatoes when you were in the middle of a tennis tournament. You wouldn't want to take much time to eat, and you certainly wouldn't want a heavy meal.

Children can't eat large volumes of food at one time, and they really prefer small amounts frequently. Recent research has shown that this is a healthier way to eat than the three squares of former days. Researchers found that eating one large meal a day caused more weight gain and raised the level of fat in the blood of adult subjects more than did the same meal divided into six parts distributed through the day. It may not seem as though children are eating enough food at any one time, but overall they're meeting their needs.

Erratic eating habits are also related to growth patterns. Jean Piaget, a distinguished French psychologist, measured linear growth and weight gain of his own children every day and found that children don't grow in an even manner. They may add a few ounces at one time, then not gain for a week or more. During the nongrowth times, they don't need to eat as much. As adults, we often eat because it's meal time, or we want a break from work, or we're bored, or it's socially required. Children listen to their bodies more than we do, and if children are not hungry, they don't need to eat.

What do you do with a baby that refuses to eat green beans or broccoli or any green vegetables you make? Well, there isn't a lot you can do. As a child, my stepson refused to eat anything green. Nothing his parents or his Auntie Beenie did could prevent him from spitting green things back or leaving them on his plate. He's a robust and healthy man in spite of that today, and now one of his favorite foods is fresh spinach with garlic and olive oil. If children refuse a certain type of food, be assured that they will eventually grow into them.

If you're really convinced that your child will develop beriberi from not eating vegetables, sneak a little puréed vegetable into some other food. However, children can usually pick up the presence of a food they hate quicker than radar. Sneak tactics can backfire and cause children to distrust even the foods they like. There are a variety of nutrients in all foods, and the absence of any single food from a child's diet won't cause nutritional problems. Picky eaters survive just as well as hearty eaters.

As for parents who cajole, coax, or try to force children to eat, guess who wins? Thc child, of course, while parents end up frustrated and angry, and the meal ends up on the floor. This is especially regrettable at dinnertime, since dinner is often the only time when parents and children sit together. It would be so nice if supper could be a peaceful, pleasant time rather than a time to monitor a two year old's broccoli intake.

Don't reward children for cleaning up what's on the plate. If you do, the message is not to stop eating when they're full, but to eat all of whatever is in front of them. Eating more than you require invariably leads to obesity.

One of my patients has six children. She said that the rule in her house is "If you don't like the food, take a bite for every year of your age." Two bites if you're only two is not hard to do. This works for her and may work for you. But if it doesn't, back off. That's how to avoid peas in your hair.

FIVE

Vitamins and Minerals

FLUORIDE AND IRON

THE BENEFICIAL ROLE of fluoride in dental health was discovered accidentally. The population in certain geographic areas had unusually low rates of dental cavities, and this was ultimately traced to the presence of fluoride in the water supply. Fluoride is incorporated into enamel as teeth develop and hardens them, making them cavity-resistant.

The fluoride in toothpaste and the flouride that dentists apply on children's teeth during dental checkups helps somewhat but isn't as effective in preventing cavities as ingesting fluoride on a daily basis through drinking water. Pediatricians are knowledgeable about the fluoride levels in their patients' water supply and will prescribe a fluoride supplement if necessary. Even if the level of fluoride in a water supply is optimum, your children need a supplement if your family only drinks plain, unfluoridated bottled water.

With well water, the fluoride level of each particular well has to be tested because some wells may contain too much fluoride for children, which causes teeth to be permanently mottled. If this is the case, children should drink bottled water.

Iron is another necessary mineral for the production of red blood cells and for the prevention of anemia. Pediatricians check a child's blood count at nine months, because this is the age when babies have depleted their iron reserves and a deficiency may first appear. After nine months, we check a child's blood count every few years.

Red meat is the best dietary source of iron. Fruits and vegetables contain iron, but they're also high in fiber, which interferes with the absorption of iron. Therefore, from the age of nine months on, infants should have two to three servings of red meat per week. Cow's milk and breast milk contain very little iron, so don't try to compensate with extra milk—you'll be giving your child an iron-deficient diet. Iron supplements should only be given on the recommendation of your doctor. Even small amount of extra iron can cause constipation and abdominal cramping. Iron is also very toxic if taken in excess, and if a toddler accidently takes the whole bottle, the results could be tragic. Therefore, have medicinal iron in the house only if absolutely necessary.

SALT AND SUGAR

We know that excessive salt intake is related to vascular disease—high blood pressure (or hypertension), heart disease, and strokes—and recent research has shown that reducing salt in childhood has a beneficial effect on later dietary habits and general health.

Dr. Forrest Adams, a pediatric cardiologist who has studied blood pressure in childhood for many years, contends that healthier populations in other parts of the world have lower average blood pressures in adulthood than we have. In America, stress, obesity, and a higher-than-necessary salt intake have raised our "average" blood pressure. Our standard of what is "normal" may actually be higher than it should be.

The effect of salt intake is cumulative: the longer high salt intake continues, the higher blood pressure will be. Therefore, the earlier in life we control salt intake, the more protection we will have against later vascular disease. Fortunately, preference for salt is an acquired taste. In a study of twins conducted by Dr. Sandra Daughtery of the University of Nevada School of Medicine, one member of each set of identical infant twins was put on a low-salt diet. When a higher salt diet was introduced, these children refused the saltier food that their twins were eating with gusto.

There is no need to add salt to anything a baby eats. Since manufacturers of baby food stopped adding salt to their products, studies have shown that homemade baby food may be *higher* in salt than commercial baby food. Parents who customarily salt water for steaming vegetables or who use salted butter add unnecessary salt to their children's diets. Therefore, commercial infant foods are at least as good as, if not better than, some homemade foods.

In the best of all possible worlds, there should be no reason for children to eat anything with added sugar! Cookies, cake, candy, and sugared drinks are high in calories, are low in other nutrients, and promote tooth decay. Also some children show a sensitivity to sugar, becoming irritable and wakeful or droopy and depressed after a sugar load.

I think sugared cereals should be taken off the market. It's all right with me when patients visit my office with little plastic bags full of Cheerios or Wheat Chex as snacks for their toddlers. But when the bags are full of Sugar Corn Pops or Cocoa Puffs, I see red. Manufactured foods must list ingredients on the package so that the major ingredient by weight appears first. Buy cereals in which sugar is at least the third ingredient listed. Granola is not necessarily better than other cereals because it's often made with a large amount of brown sugar, which is no better than white.

SUPPLEMENTARY VITAMINS

Infants and toddlers in this country receive more vitamins than they need. Breast milk contains both vitamins and transport factors, substances that enhance the absorption of vitamins, and vitamins are added to commercial formula. Vitamin supplements are routinely added to milk, cereal, and other foods. Vitamins are not foods themselves, but enzymes that function in the metabolism of food. Humans cannot store extra vitamins, so daily excess is disposed of through urine and feces. This prompted one of my instructors in medical school to say, "The urine of American children is the most nutritious in the world."

I don't think healthy, normal children need extra vitamins. The only exception might be children who live in cold climates with long winters who are not exposed to sunlight for long periods. If you feel compelled to use vitamins, be aware of their drawbacks. Manufacturers add flavorings, sweeteners, and coloring agents to liquid vitamins to make them palatable, and any of these can have side effects; buy a kind without artificial color or flavoring. Buy the cheapest you can find—the vitamins at a health-food store are exactly the same as those at a discount drug store. Also, if your child refuses them, don't fight about it. It's not worth it.

There are absolutely no—I repeat, no—vitamins that are safe to take in large doses (this applies equally to children and adults). High doses of vitamin C taken over several months, for example, interfere with the absorption of copper, important to the normal functioning of the nervous system. Recently, a patient was giving her son high doses of vitamin C as well as aspirin for his cold. I had to put the little boy in the hospital when the combination of vitamin C and aspirin burned the lining of his stomach enough to make it bleed.

DIETARY SUPPLEMENTS

At a routine exam, the mother of a one year old asked me what I thought about substituting a drink with a strange name for milk. Since her child hadn't shown any signs of intolerance to milk, I wondered why she wanted to change.

"The woman who sells it convinced me that it would be better than milk," she said. When I said I thought it unwise to be convinced by someone making money from the sale of the product, she countered, "I know that there are people out there trying to make money, but this woman is selling it at her own cost!"

Dietary supplements have not been subjected to any type of rigorous scientific testing. Their manufacturers deny that they have any deleterious effects, but the American Academy of Pediatrics recently issued a statement after examining some of the milk substitutes available. It found them *all* to be nutritionally inadequate and inappropriate for children.

Interactions of dietary elements are very complex, and manufacturers of cockamamie products are giving consumers simplistic, incorrect answers to complicated problems and are making a lot of money while doing it. Take the money you would have spent on vitamins and dietary supplements, and buy fresh strawberries in winter or some other healthy treat for your family. Remember that a variety of fresh, unprocessed, unsalted food is an ideal diet for babies as well as adults. And take any nutritional advice you receive from suspect sources with a grain of salt substitute.

Health foods are not healthier foods. There is nothing about an apple bought in a health-food store that is any better or different from an apple bought at a supermarket, although it is more expensive. The *Journal of the American Dietetic Association* reported that food from health-food stores costs significantly more than the same food from a supermarket, yet there is no difference in pesticide levels nor in nutritional content.

Remember also that parents play a significant role in their children's nutrition by what the adults themselves eat. Children imitate what parents do, not what they say. The choices you make about your own diet are important, too. If you follow the basic rules of common sense and feed your child a reasonable variety of fresh foods, your baby will be well nourished and feeding your child will be a joy.

SIX

Visiting the Doctor: Well-Baby Visits and Immunization

IN THE FIRST two years of your child's life you'll be making frequent visits to your pediatrician's office for regular checkups and immunization shots as well as for minor illnesses. This is the best part of pediatrics for me, because I get to know the babies and their parents and watch them all grow together.

Most pediatricians see babies more often in the first few months, with visits gradually decreasing over the first two years. Typically, I examine an infant a day or two after hospital discharge to check the weight, to see that the baby isn't jaundiced, that the parents are comfortable, and that breast feeding is going well. Subsequent visits are at two weeks, once a month to six months, then at three-month intervals. During the next year, visits will be when the child is fifteen months, eighteen months, and two years.

We call these regular visits "well-baby visits." Their purpose is to measure physical growth, to be alert to any congenital problems early, to assess development, to educate and assist parents, and to obtain immunizations.

Nurses or medical assistants will weigh the baby and measure length and head circumference at each well-check. At the baby's first visit, you may learn that your baby has shrunk! An infant who was twenty inches long at birth may register 19½ inches in the pediatrician's office. Muscle tone is lax at birth, so the baby is more easily measured. As muscle tone increases, the baby's length will appear to be shorter.

An infant's weight gain in the first two months may be as much as an ounce a day. Weight doubles by six months, then the rate of gain lessens by the age of one year and is even slower after that. Formerly, parents nearly always asked me if a baby was gaining weight fast enough, but today's weight-conscious parents now ask if their baby is gaining too fast!

As a rule, breast-fed babies gain more slowly than bottle-fed babies. Pediatricians are aware of this, and we often prevent a supplementary bottle from being added unnecessarily when babies gain a little slowly.

Congenital problems and minor malformations are rare, but the earlier they're diagnosed, the easier they are to treat. For example, you'll see your pediatrician manipulate baby's legs and hips and check the symmetry of the buttocks. The reason for this maneuver is to check for shallow hip sockets, a condition called "congenital dislocation of the hips." This is more common in babies who were delivered in breech position or those with a family history of this problem, but the condition can appear in any child.

If there is congenital dislocation, walking is delayed, gait is abnormal, and the hip joint may degenerate in later life. Surgery may then be necessary. If the condition is diagnosed in infancy, however, all that is needed is a simple brace for a few months to encourage normal hip development. This condition may or may not have been apparent at birth, so periodic examinations are necessary to insure early diagnosis. I often discover such easily solved problems at a routine visit, and this prevents later complications.

Pediatricians regularly reassure parents that their child's development is normal. If, by chance, a developmental problem should exist, studies show that the earlier special intervention begins, the better the outcome, so pediatricians watch closely to intervene early with developmental deviations. Most metropolitan areas have preschool programs, public and private, for children with special needs.

Daniel was not yet saying single words by eighteen months and was a distractible, seemingly hyperactive child. Between his delayed speech and poor performance in areas of development requiring concentration, he was labeled possibly retarded and/or autistic. However, diligent investigation showed that he had a profound hearing loss. Deaf children, of course, will not speak, and his behavior was difficult to control because he couldn't hear his parents' commands. Once he was fitted for hearing aids and his parents learned to attract his attention more effectively, his behavior improved and his development advanced by leaps and bounds.

Parents should leave the well-baby visit feeling that they've learned something. You should know what to expect in your child's development in the next few months, know how to advance your child's diet, know what safety tips are relevant to the child's age, and have some advance information about health problems you may encounter such as fever or diarrhea. In my practice we give parents information sheets about fever, vomiting, and diarrhea at routine visits.

The time your doctor spends may vary—from five to perhaps twenty minutes, depending on what you need and want. I find that mothers tend to be consistent from visit to visit: one mother will always have a list of several questions, and another will always seem content just to know her baby is doing well. What's important is that you feel the doctor has listened to you and has answered all your questions. If you want more time, ask for it, and don't let the doctor leave until you're satisfied.

If you have an urgent question, you should feel free to telephone at any time; but write routine questions down as they occur to you, and bring them along to your appointment. Also, some of the most significant questions I've been asked over the years are the "by the ways" that patients mention as my hand is on the door.

Sometimes I try an experiment with a new parent. At four months, if the baby is doing very well and the parents seem confident, I'll suggest that we skip the next month's visit and see each other in two months. More often than not, parents want to come in anyway, showing me how important the visits can be.

The final reason for regular visits is immunization. Parents invariably say that they thought measles has been eradicated, so why are we giving the shot? Ever since the World Health Organization announced the world-wide eradication of smallpox, people think that the other preventable diseases such as measles, diphtheria, polio, mumps, tetanus, rubella, and whooping cough have also been eliminated. Unfortunately, that's not true. Smallpox is a unique disease that was conquered over a period of thirty years as the result of a world-wide cooperative effort. Once it was eradicated, the risk of side effects from the vaccine became greater than the risk of contracting the disease and the immunization was no longer given. But such is not the case with other childhood diseases.

The diseases we currently immunize children against are commonplace all over the world and are major causes of infant mortality. Because of emigration from countries where the diseases are epidemic and mass travel to all parts of the world, there is still considerable risk.

American parents see these diseases rarely, if at all, *because* American children are immunized. Without immunization, widespread epidemics would likely occur. This happened in Japan and England when controversy over pertussis (whooping cough) vaccine prompted parents and doctors to withhold immunization. Shortly thereafter there were tens of thousands of cases of pertussis, leading to hundreds of deaths and hospitalizations.

The controversy over risks of immunization in this country arose in April 1982 when two highly inaccurate national television programs sensationalized the possible adverse consequences of the pertussis immunization. These shows stated that serious complications resulting from the vaccine were as high as 1 in 700, when the actual rate of serious side effects is 1 in 310,000 to 500,000. For a child who is not immunized and who contracts the infection, the rate of serious complications is 1 in 10,000. So the risk of the disease is many times more dangerous than side effects from the vaccine. There have been numerous articles and books endeavoring to convince parents that immunizations are not only unnecessary but harmful. With all my heart I say that the risk is minuscule compared with the threat of the diseases.

I'll review the immunizations, the rare side effects, and the circumstances under which some shots should not be given. As a general rule, we don't administer any shot to a child who has an infection, especially if there is a fever.

DIPHTHERIA, PERTUSSIS (WHOOPING COUGH), AND TETANUS

Most children will have minor reactions to this shot (known as DPT immunization). These may include fever, fretfulness, or soreness at the place of the injection, usually the upper leg in infants. Sometimes the area of injection becomes red and swollen. A lump may appear and persist for several weeks, although tenderness subsides in a day or two. Fever as high as 101 degrees may last for a few hours. If your child's temperature rises over 101, and especially if it lasts more than a few hours, consult your pediatrician. The pertussis part of the vaccine is the major cause of reactions; if prolonged fever occurs, the diphtheria-tetanus portion of the shot without the pertussis part may be the choice for the future. Your pediatrician should also know if your child cries for longer than an hour or two after the shot, or becomes pale and faint and is difficult to arouse within a few moments. Children with certain neurological diseases and those who experienced previous side effects from the diphtheria-pertussis-tetanus vaccine should not receive the pertussis fraction.

We still have much to learn in medicine, but we know that nothing in medicine is or ever will be 100-percent effective. Although 10 to 15 percent of immunized children can still contract whooping cough, the course of the disease will be considerably milder and complications less likely if immunization has taken place.

The tetanus fraction of the DPT vaccine can cause some pain and soreness at the place of injection, but allergic reactions are rare and occur exclusively in older children and adults. Since tetanus carries a statistic of 50-percent mortality even today, there should be no question of the necessity and efficacy of the shot. Tetanus-producing bacteria are present not only in the soil but even in the mouths of humans and animals, and for those not immunized the possibility of contracting the disease is great.

Diphtheria is a deadly disease, but the vaccine has virtually no toxicity. In 1982 there were only two cases of diphtheria in the United States, but there are thousands of cases elsewhere in the world. Therefore, we continue to give the injection along with tetanus throughout childhood.

A few years ago, Dr. Larry Baroff and his colleagues at UCLA published a study suggesting that the DPT vaccine may be associated with sudden infant death syndrome, or crib death. Many people remember this and still ask me about it. Four subsequent studies, including a large-scale, multicenter national study, showed no such association.

Since the DPT shot can cause pain and fever immediately after injection, I give mothers in my office a small sample of acetaminophen drops (Tempra, Tylenol, Panadol, etc.) to ease their babies' discomfort.

POLIO

In my own childhood, polio epidemics struck fear in the hearts of parents each summer. Before the vaccine was introduced, there were 24,000 cases of polio in this country in a single year; a few years later, after widespread use of the vaccine, only 20 cases. The original vaccine developed by Jonas Salk was an injection of killed viruses, but the more recently developed Sabin vaccine is a live, weakened virus given by mouth. The oral form has great advantages. Not only is injection by needle unnecessary, but ingestion of the virus into the gastrointestinal tract confers an additional measure of immunity by causing antibodies to form in the intestine.

The polio vaccine has no known side effects, but make sure that all adults in your household have been vaccinated. There is a slight risk of transmitting the virus to susceptible adults. The risk of a healthy person contracting polio from the vaccine, however, is minuscule—about 1 in 4 million doses. Children whose immunity is impaired, such as those under treatment for cancer or kidney transplantation, should not receive polio or any other live-virus vaccines.

MEASLES

The vaccine for measles was introduced to the United States in the 1960s, and the number of cases decreased to a record low in 1982. Proof of immunization is required when a child enters elementary school, and 95 percent of children entering school since 1980–1981 are now immunized. There are many areas in the world, however, where the major cause of infant mortality is measles. A devastating encephalitis can occur in as many as 4 out of 1,000 children with the infection; the vaccine, on the other hand, may cause encephalitis in 1 out of 1 million doses. Compare that to the risk of the disease, and there can be no question that the benefits of immunization far outweigh the risks.

Some children do have a minor local reaction consisting of redness and swelling for a day or two at the site of injection, and others may have a slight fever and rash for from seven to fourteen days after the shot.

As with polio and all live-virus vaccines, the measles vaccine should not be given to any child with a disorder that suppresses immune responses. There have been no reports of measles being transmitted by the vaccine from immunized children to susceptible contacts.

MUMPS

Mumps is an infection characterized by swelling of the parotid or salivary glands on the sides of the face near the ears. Parents often think that a child with swollen lymph nodes has mumps, but they're usually wrong. Mumps can also infect the brain, acoustic nerve, pancreas, and testicles, causing deafness, a life-threatening pancreatitis, and, in rare cases, sterility.

The mumps vaccine was licensed in 1968 and was almost immediately incorporated into the MMR (measles, mumps, and rubella) shot. In 1977 the incidence of mumps had dropped from prevaccine levels of tens of thousands of cases per year to 20,000, and by 1982 there were about 5,000 cases annually. The incidence of mumps in those states where mumps immunization is not required for school entry is about twice as high as in those where immunization is prescribed by law.

The vaccine is given at fifteen months along with the vaccination for measles, mumps, and rubella, and there are no significant side effects.

RUBELLA

Rubella—more popularly known as German or three-day measles—has two forms. It can be an acute brief viral illness that is one of the most benign of childhood diseases, causing only a mild fever, a slight rash, and illness for three days. But when the virus infects a pregnant woman, its effect on the developing fetus is less benign. Depending on the stage of pregnancy during which the mother is infected and the severity of the infection, congenital rubella can cause heart defects, mental retardation, and deafness in the infant. Two years after birth, 80 percent of infants born to mothers infected with rubella during pregnancy will be affected. Therefore, it's essential (1) that all women be immunized by childbearing age and (2) that the reservoir of rubella in the community be eliminated, which is the reason that we immunize male children as well.

Since the introduction of rubella vaccine in 1969, there has been a 96-percent decrease in the incidence of the disease. Before the vaccine was introduced, tens of thousands of cases of congenital rubella were reported following an epidemic in 1964. In 1982 there were just seven cases of congenital rubella, and twenty in 1983.

The rubella vaccine, like the disease it's preventing, can cause transient joint pain, more commonly if given to adolescents or adults than to infants. This is only a temporary inflammation and has nothing to do with later arthritis.

It will take from ten to thirty years before the children we are immunizing today will reach childbearing age. At that time, congenital rubella may have disappeared in this country. Until then, we have an obligation to future generations to immunize our children today.

H. FLU VACCINE

The major serious infectious disease that pediatricians treat is that caused by *Haemophilus influenzae*, or H. flu. This has nothing to do with the viral flu that goes around all winter. H. Flu, is a bacterium that causes serious disease in small children—meningitis and epiglottitis—as well as less serious ones such as middle ear infections. A vaccine became available in mid-1985 that appears safe and effective, and is given to children at two years of age. If children are in day care, they should receive it at eighteen months.

SCHEDULE OF IMMUNIZATION

The schedule of immunizations is as follows:

2 months . . .	DPT and polio
4 months . . .	DPT and polio
6 months . . .	DPT and polio
15 months . . .	MMR
18 months . . .	DPT and polio
2 years . . .	H. flu
4 to 6 years . . .	DPT and polio

Every ten years after that, the tetanus shot should be administered.

You needn't remember the schedule—your pediatrician should tell you when the next shot is due—but keep a record of the shots your child receives. Your doctor or the clinic staff will give you a wallet-sized card or small book which should be updated with each shot. Store this in a safe place. When your child enters school, proof of immunization is required.

Sometimes a child's schedule of immunizations is interrupted by illness, parental forgetfulness, or the fact that the family has moved. If there is a long delay between immunizations, we don't have to start all over again but can resume the schedule where we left off.

Many new mothers wince and say something like "I've been dreading this all week" when I tell them it's time to start their baby's shots. Of course, it hurts, and, yes, some babies are uncomfortable for a few hours afterward. But if you approach it as a necessary discomfort for an ultimately greater good and an opportunity to help your child cope with the first of many minor stresses, the upset will be minimized for both you and your baby.

Sometimes, no matter how carefully we prepare children, we just can't do enough. Mercedes needed to have two tiny stitches removed from her cheek where the emergency-room doctor had mended a small cut. Coincidentally, I had a small mole removed a few days before from the very same spot. I had two-year-old Mercedes sitting on my chest watching closely as my partner removed my stitches while I made elaborate comments on how much fun it was and how it didn't hurt. When it was her turn, however, we still needed two adults to keep her still while I removed her tear-washed stitches.

Newborns in a nursery who were encouraged to suck on a pacifier before, during, and after a needle prick cried less and quieted down sooner than babies without pacifiers. This simply confirms what we already know: if someone or something helps us through a painful ordeal, it will be easier. One of my mothers whose son was about to receive a shot said softly to him, "I know you're not going to like this. You're going to feel a pain in your leg. It's a shot, and afterwards you're probably going to cry. But I'll pick you up and give you a big hug." Her four month old couldn't understand her words, but the message was entirely clear; in a soothing tone she was reassuring him that she would help him through a somewhat unpleasant experience. Close contact while the shot is being administered and hugging and comforting immediately afterward can minimize the discomfort.

Mothers who ask to leave the room because they can't bear to see pain are certainly entitled to leave, but I try to convince them that it would be better to stay. Toddlers who are old enough to understand should be told that they're going to have a shot and that it will hurt a little. I shouldn't have to tell you not to say that the shot won't hurt—it will. But telling a child it will hurt for a second and will then be over is realistic and helpful.

VACCINES AND THE FUTURE

Although effective, the pertussis vaccine for whooping cough has the highest rate of complications and side effects. Research centers in several countries are working on an improved vaccine. Research trials in Japan suggest that a new vaccine causes far less fever and local side effects. However, since the new Japanese vaccine has only been tried on a few thousand children and the long-term side effects are not yet known, it may take a few years before the vaccine receives approval in the United States.

Researchers world-wide are also working on a chickenpox vaccine, and again Japanese research seems to be in the forefront. Chickenpox is a tricky virus, but we may see a vaccine in general use within the next year or two.

Fear of vaccine side effects and reluctance to have their children immunized were aroused in parents because of the publicity surrounding lawsuits brought by the parents of children who suffered serious side effects of vaccination. The tragedy of even one life harmed cannot be minimized, but the slight possibility of harm must be weighed against the risks of ceasing immunizations altogether.

If states require shots for school entrance and, more importantly, if it's our public-health obligation to have our children immunized, then society should take responsibility for the rare adverse consequences. In 1983, Senator Paula Hawkins (R–Florida) introduced a bill into the Senate called the

National Child Vaccination–Injury Compensation Act, which would permit prompt, equitable compensation for the few children injured by immunization. Monies for the compensation fund would be provided by a surcharge on each dose of vaccine. The American Academy of Pediatrics has been working toward implementing this program.

The ideal vaccine would be one that confers 100-percent immunity with no side effects. Unfortunately, there has never been and never will be such a thing. There is always the risk of potential complication to any intervention, whether by shots, drugs, or herbs. But I hope I've convinced you that the risks of the diseases far outweigh the risks of the vaccines.

SEVEN

On-the-Job Training: The First Weeks with Your Baby

THE FIRST WEEKS with a newborn in the house are exciting and wonderful, but, as parents soon realize, it's on-the-job training twenty-four hours a day. Many questions arise as parents and newborns are getting to know each other. Some can be answered easily (with reassurance and a prescription for common sense); others take a little more time.

In this chapter, I will cover the topics that parents most often ask me about in the office and on the phone. The first section deals with the home environment and the daily activities of bathing, diapering, and sleep. These are the issues that are common to all new parents. Next, I'll take up less frequent concerns, such as nighttime waking and what to do about pacifiers. Finally, I've included a brief description of some minor medical conditions that babies may develop in the first few weeks of life.

If you have further questions, you shouldn't hesitate or be embarrassed to call your pediatrician. However, the material in this chapter may save you an unnecessary visit to the doctor's office.

SETTLING DOWN AT HOME (AND GOING OUT)

As they leave the hospital for the variable temperatures of the outside world, many parents wrap their babies as though they were about to take a day-long journey in a Russian snowstorm. Once home, they also have a tendency to keep the baby bundled up and to overheat the house. It's true that babies can lose body heat and develop a chill more quickly than adults, but they're not hothouse orchids. Your house or apartment should be about 72 degrees Fahrenheit, a temperature that is comfortable for everyone. A baby should be dressed as heavily or lightly as you are. If the indoor temperature is 75 degrees and you're wearing a cotton T-shirt and shorts, your baby doesn't need seventeen layers of clothing. Parents often consult me about puzzling fevers that are "cured" once I remove excess clothing.

At cool temperatures, your baby's skin takes on a mottled bluish color (called *cutis marmorata,* or marble skin). This is caused by constriction of the superficial blood vessels and only means that your child needs another blanket or a pair of socks.

The indoor air of a house or apartment is usually dry, which causes the mucus in the nose and throat of babies to thicken. Since newborns can't sniff or blow their noses or clear their throats, they often sound as if they have a cold. This congestion usually bothers parents more than it does babies. If the air in your house is dry, use a humidifier while the baby sleeps to provide the necessary moisture.

Before you left the hospital, you may have received a soft plastic bulb syringe for removing mucus from the baby's nose. Usually, these are not very effective, and repeated attempts to aspirate mucus will only irritate a newborn's delicate nasal membranes. Also, this procedure hurts (try it on yourself). My advice is don't upset a baby who seems content, and use the syringe only to remove mucus that is visible.

While you're settling in at home, it's not a good idea to have frequent visitors. Your new schedule may be all that you can handle, and guests will interfere with your rest and routines. When people who aren't immediate family call to ask when they can see the baby, give them a definite date, but make it in a week or two.

No sooner are parents settled in a home with their new baby than they ask how soon they can take the baby out. Leaving home with a baby is no simple matter and requires planning—you can no longer grab your purse and go. The diaper bag must be filled; an extra outfit must be chosen in case the baby spits up or diapers leak; the baby must be changed and dressed, bottles filled, and so forth. Often, parents with a new baby are late for their first appointment at my office, and I'm never surprised or angry.

New parents are even more likely to overdress their babies for outdoors than they do for indoors. On outside jaunts, dress the baby appropriately for the season, but don't hesitate to plan a brief change of scene. On a pleasant day, even if there's a nip in the air, the fresh air will do you both good, even if it's only a walk around the block or a sojourn in the backyard.

Until the age of four weeks, pediatricians recommend that you avoid large groups of people or any group of small children because newborns are extremely susceptible to certain infections. Visits to Grandma's house and small private outings are fine.

THE INS AND OUTS OF BELLY BUTTONS

In the hospital nursery, an infant's umbilical cord is usually treated to prevent infection, often with a blue substance called Triple Dye. After three or four days, the umbilical remnant, by then dark brown or black in color, is usually dry and shrivels up.

The remnant of the umbilical cord may remain attached for several weeks or may detach itself within one week. The area should be kept dry until it does. Let air circulate by folding the diaper to expose the navel. Sponge bathe the baby until the cord detaches, since an accumulation of water beneath the cord can promote infection. You can hasten the drying of the cord by applying to it rubbing alcohol with a cotton swab or a piece of gauze whenever you change the diaper.

When the umbilical remnant detaches, a small amount of bright red blood may be apparent for a day or two. If you see a blood spot on the baby's diaper, keep the navel exposed and be sure the area is absolutely dry. If there is a secretion of clear or yellowish fluid and a small gray or light brown bump inside the navel, an umbilical granuloma may have formed. This is simply an overgrowth of tissue that forms as the navel heals. Your pediatrician can cauterize the area with some silver nitrate. The procedure is painless.

If the skin around your baby's navel is inflamed or if there is odor, consult your pediatrician. Infections in and around the navel can become serious. We treat infections in that area vigorously with antibiotics and watch the baby carefully for signs of a systemic infection.

After the navel heals, most babies have an "innie," a belly button that looks like a little cup. However, in some children there is a minor weakness in the abdominal-wall musculature, and when the navel heals they are left with an "outie," or an umbilical hernia. An umbilical hernia is not caused by the way the cord was cut—the condition was present before the baby was born.

Uneccessary and unsanitary home remedies have been devised to treat umbilical hernias. These range from special binders to taping a twenty-five-cent piece over the hernia. None of these is recommended. Anything applied to a baby's skin for any period of time will cause skin breakdown and infections. As far as binders are concerned, they may be too tight and restrict a baby's breathing.

An umbilical hernia is a condition that will likely right itself in a few years. If your child is one of the very few who still has an outie by the age of ten and is bothered by this, the condition can be surgically corrected. Surgery at that age is safer and less traumatic than it is for an infant.

BATHING: HOW MUCH IS TOO MUCH?

Newborns really don't need to be bathed every day. Every two or three days are enough. Babies don't perspire, they don't play in the mud, and they aren't eating peanut-butter and jelly sandwiches. Besides, we probably bathe too much in this country. Personal hygiene is important, of course, but small babies only need to have their mouths and chins sponged and the diaper area attended to.

Babies who are bathed too often have dry, itchy, scaly

skin. Water itself removes surface oils that help retain moisture. The creams and lotions that many people use to try to restore moisture often contain alcohol and water, which may cause further drying. If your baby still has dry skin, even when bathed every two or three days, I suggest using Keri lotion or Eucerin cream. Your own pediatrician may have a favorite brand to recommend.

Until the umbilical cord detaches and the navel is dry, newborns should be sponge-bathed rather than submerged in a bath.

When it's time for a real bath, you can bathe the baby either in the tub or in the sink. The kitchen sink as a bathing area is kinder to parents' backs. Babies are slippery when they're wet, and new parents may feel safer if they set the baby in a plastic laundry basket in the water. A spongy, water-absorbent pad will also provide security, and there are bath rings especially manufactured to support and hold a child. These can be found in stores that carry equipment for children.

Before immersing your baby, draw the water in the tub or sink, and check the temperature with your wrist or elbow; your hand alone is not sensitive enough to gauge whether the water is too hot.

Some mothers and fathers like to take their babies into the tub with them. If you want to do this—and I personally think this is a lovely, intimate way for parents to enjoy close contact with their babies—test the water carefully with your wrist or elbow. Place a towel on the floor beside the tub, set the baby down, and climb in yourself. Once you're in a secure sitting position, reach over and lift the baby in with you. When you're finished, reverse the procedure: place the baby on the towel beside the tub before climbing out.

Whatever bathing method you use, all supplies should be

within easy reach before you bring the baby to the bath. Never leave a child alone in the water—even for a moment. Let the phone ring, and ignore the doorbell. An unattended child can drown in one inch of water.

You can use a mild soap such as Johnson & Johnson baby soap, Neutrogena, or castile soap, or put a drop or two of Alpha Keri oil in the bath water instead of soap. Actually, soap can make the baby slippery as well as dry out the skin, so it's all right to bathe the baby in clear water alone.

Wash the baby gently with a soft cloth, and be sure to clean all the crevices such as inside the folds of the neck. Afterward, be sure that all those little crevices are dry, too. The baby's hair need only be washed about once a week. Use the same soap that was used for the body, or use a mild baby shampoo.

All babies don't feel the same way about being bathed. Some relax happily and love being washed, and others loathe the experience and object to it from the moment they're undressed until they're dressed again. If bathing is not a happy time for your child, don't force the issue: make do with a quick sponge bath, and have a full bath once a week.

In the past, mothers used to powder their babies after a bath on the theory that powder absorbed moisture and would prevent rashes and irritation. However, we no longer subscribe to that notion. I once helped care for a child with severe recurrent asthma. Whenever he was discharged from the hospital, he'd be back in a day or two. We tested him for every allergy and sensitivity, and even explored the possibility of psychological problems between the mother and child. The mystery was solved when he was examined at home, where baby powder was found to be causing his "allergy." Many children, like this little boy, have an extreme sensitivity to baby powder. Some children may have bouts of wheezing; others may develop only mild, coldlike symptoms. This child was never powdered in the hospital, and once his mother stopped powdering him at home, he never had to return to the hospital.

Pediatricians, including myself, advise against baby powder. Even cornstarch has its drawbacks: although it's not likely to emit particles, cornstarch is a wonderful medium for growth of the fungus that causes diaper rash. The new paper diapers are so absorbent, there's really no need for extra powder in the diaper area. Dry your baby well when you change diapers and after the bath, and you probably won't have to worry about rashes or respiratory problems.

If your home has its own water heater, make sure the temperature is not set higher than 110 degrees Fahrenheit or the medium setting on the gauge. Older children can turn on water taps, and tender baby skin scalds easily in just a second or two if water is over 120 degrees. If you live in an apartment and can't set the temperature gauge, be very careful whenever you turn on the hot-water faucets.

DIAPERS AND ELIMINATION

Parents focus much attention on elimination and spend a lot of time changing diapers. The first question I'm asked is whether to use cloth or paper diapers. In my practice, I see a zillion paper diapers to one cloth diaper. Cloth diapers are certainly less expensive, although the difference in cost is not as great as it may seem. There's not only the cost of the diapers themselves, but the cost of the detergent, running the washer and dryer, the cost of the diaper service if you use one, and the cost of your own time rinsing out cloth diapers and soaking them. And nothing beats the convenience of paper diapers. Nearly all the mothers I know use them when their babies are outside the home.

Neither type of diaper is intrinsically better or worse as far as babies are concerned, although paper diapers are now being made with materials that are extremely absorbent. These draw moisture effectively away from the baby's skin, preventing rashes and bacterial growth. As to comfort, some babies are sensitive to the fibers in paper diapers, and some are sensitive to the residual chemicals in cloth ones. Use whichever one seems to suit your baby.

In the first twenty-four to forty-eight hours of life, babies' stools are tarry, black-green in color and have no odor. After two or three days, stools become mustard yellow and either seedy, watery, or a combination of the two. Some babies evacuate every time they eat, others have a stool every three or four days. The laxative companies have made us think that regularity is a virtue, but some people are naturally regular and some are not. As long as your baby seems comfortable and is taking nourishment, don't worry about the frequency or regularity of bowel movements.

At first, parents discover that the baby has had a bowel movement by finding it in the diaper. By one month of age, however, babies start to grunt, strain, turn red in the face, and even cry when they have a stool. Understandably, parents may assume that this is due to constipation. Actually, the baby is just starting to participate more in the act of elimination. As long as the stool is soft, there's no cause for concern. Just as some babies love being bathed and some don't, some babies feel pleasure in moving their bowels and others don't.

Breast-fed babies may have small, frequent stools or one stool every few days, but they are always watery and sometimes a little seedy. Formula-fed babies have less frequent and slightly harder stools. As new foods are introduced, the character and frequency of stools change. For example, some babies will pass harder stools after they start to eat rice cereal. If more solid stools are painful and difficult to pass, give the baby extra water. For greater palatability, you might sweeten the water with a little dark Karo syrup, a small amount of prune juice, or blackstrap molasses. But because of the association between honey and infant botulism, don't sweeten the water with honey until the baby is over one year old. When the baby is four to six months old, purèed prunes or baby prune juice may help to loosen the stools.

Cow's milk may cause constipation. If you find that your child passes hard and infrequent stools shortly after starting to drink cow's milk, eliminate the milk to see if the condition improves. Your pediatrician can recommend a substitute for cow's milk if this is the problem.

If your baby has stools that are too firm, don't administer enemas or use suppositories without first consulting your pediatrician. Such solutions can be harmful under certain circumstances and may foster a dependency on mechanical aids for elimination.

The color of stool sometimes concerns parents. Not a week goes by that I don't receive a call asking about the green color of a stool. This may be caused by a small amount of bile that wasn't digested thoroughly or simply because the baby ate spinach or green Jell-O. Green stools are normal and are no cause for concern.

In contrast to the variable frequency of bowel movements, babies must urinate frequently. Pediatricians are particularly aware of how often babies urinate because we remove so many diapers each day and suffer the consequences so directly.

Babies usually have a very dilute, light yellow urine and

wet their diapers at least six or eight times a day. In the first week or two, a transient high concentration of a certain amino acid may cause the urine to be pink, and parents may mistake this for blood. If your baby has a pinkish-colored urine, save the diaper and ask your pediatrician if he or she wants to test it for blood. If the pink color appears only once or twice, it's probably due to this amino acid.

An inevitable consequence of diapers is diaper rash. The new improved paper diapers that have a double band of elastic around the legs, as well as cloth diapers with a layer of plastic pants over them, retain moisture and keep air out, promoting rashes. Since any skin area will become irritated and possibly infected if constantly wet and airtight, the best prevention and treatment for diaper rash is to expose the skin for a few hours each day, preferably outdoors. If weather doesn't permit this, try to keep the diaper loose.

There's no need for plastic pants over paper diapers, and if you use cloth, leave the plastic pants off when you're at home. The likelihood of diaper rash increases in the watertight environment of diapers covered by plastic.

When I was first in practice, I volunteered to babysit for a couple who were going out of town for a weekend. My friends told me that Charlie had diaper rash, and they showed me the cream they were using to help clear up the rash. After my friends left, Charlie and I spent a lot of time in the backyard, and gradually Charlie's diapers would come off. I had never put on a diaper that didn't immediately sag and fall off, probably because I put them on too loosely. When my friends returned, lo and behold Charlie's rash had disappeared.

At the time I couldn't take credit for the solution. Later I learned that in some African societies, palm leaves are the solution to diapering; when the leaf is soiled, it's replaced with a new one. Since we don't rely on palm leaves and babies can't be toilet-trained for at least two years, the next best thing is plenty of air exposure and changing diapers as soon as they are wet.

SLEEP AND SLEEPING ARRANGEMENTS

Parents often ask my advice about where a child should sleep. In a way, the answer to that question is paradoxical. If we want to do things the "natural way," it's certainly not natural to expect a baby who has been sheltered inside a mother's body to adjust immediately to spending the night alone. Also, parents newly bonded to their babies may prefer the closeness of the same room and the security of being there if the baby awakens and cries. But there are persuasive reasons for not having babies in the parental bedroom. Parents need a place to retreat from the twenty-four-hour demands of an infant, and they are better able to relax and enjoy their child if the bedroom remains their private place.

My compromise is to keep the baby in the bedroom with you for the first few weeks if this makes you feel more secure. The baby can be moved to a separate room as soon as you're comfortable doing so. Don't worry that you won't hear the baby if he or she needs you. Parents soon develop a kind of radar, and even a tiny whimper from the next room can awaken them from a deep sleep.

When babies sleep, they snort, sniffle, wheeze, whimper, and awaken slightly. New parents who aren't accustomed to these nocturnal symphonies may respond to every sound the baby makes. Too frequent attention paid to a baby who seems to need your presence to return to sleep may lead to later sleep problems. When babies awaken, they need to learn to use their own resources to fall asleep again.

Being born is a long, hard journey, and newborns may take awhile to wake up and smell the roses. They sleep more in the first twenty-four to forty-eight hours than they ever will later. After that, the amount and pattern of sleep will vary according to the baby's own personality and needs, and may be different for each baby. New parents who say "My baby doesn't sleep enough" or "My baby sleeps too much" seem to forget that when infants need to sleep, they do. If they don't need it, nothing you can do will put them to sleep. Just as some adults need seven and a half hours of sleep a night and others can manage on four hours, babies also have their individual rhythms. As a general rule, a newborn sleeps a lot, a one month old somewhat less, and a six month old is awake most of the day.

To a certain extent, babies can adapt their sleep schedules to any adult way of life. A friend of mine is an artist who had never arisen earlier than 11 A.M. before her baby was born. She asked me, "What am I going to do when he wakes up at five A.M.? All babies do that, don't they?"

I said, "Put him to bed at midnight." So she did that right from the start, and the baby consistently slept well until 9 A.M. That schedule seemed to work out for this mother and baby, although I wouldn't advise it as a general rule. Usually, parents find themselves adapting their schedules to their baby's needs.

For this reason, pediatricians advise that babies should be sleeping alone regularly by the age of six months. Does this mean that your baby should be banished from your bed after the first few weeks or months? I don't believe there's an absolute rule here, although some authorities maintain that a child should not be taken into bed for the occasional night or series of nights when he or she is fussing, teething, upset, or just lonely. Dr. Spock, whom I admire, goes so far as to say that a child should never be taken into the parents' bed.

However, according to a recent survey, 95 percent of parents said they did bring their children under five into bed with them occasionally. It's a great comfort to my patients when I tell them that almost everyone does this (they just don't talk about it) and that there are times when it's the right thing to do.

For example, a friend told me about an experience with her two-year-old daughter Amy when they were separated in a department store. After a frantic half-hour search, security personnel reunited Amy with her mother. After that incident, Amy wanted to sleep with her mother. The mother asked my advice because she'd heard that she shouldn't permit this. I felt that both mother and child had been through a scary experience. What could possibly be wrong with giving each other comfort when they needed it? (After a few nights, Amy voluntarily returned to her own bed.) As I told my friend, if it feels good to you and your child, it's probably the right thing to do.

The same goes for the family sleeping together. A few years ago when I was on a radio talk show, a mother called in to ask my opinion about the "family bed." I told her that I had once thought it was a bad practice since this was what I was taught in medical school. I then told her that I now feel if everyone is happy with the arrangement, it can't be harmful. The caller said that she had been warned that her daughter would never want to leave her parents' bed. I suggested that the mother cross that bridge when she came to it.

I heard from this mother again on a later program when her child was two and a half. The child had recently decided that it was time to have her own bed and had transferred easily to a junior bed. My point is that a "family bed" may not be right for everyone, but it can be a wonderful arrangement for those who enjoy it.

There is only one prohibition when the family sleeps together. Parents should not engage in sexual activity if children are in the same room. Children often perceive the act as hostile or harmful, and psychologists believe that lasting trauma can result. Parents who sleep with their children should find other places and times for sexual activity.

Babies traditionally sleep in cribs, but until a child is two or three months old you may only need a portacrib or cradle. If you inherit a crib or buy one that has been used before, be sure that the sides work smoothly and that there are no sharp or broken parts. Chapter Nine on safety contains more tips on what to look for when buying a crib.

A crib is a reliable and secure sleeping accommodation until your baby is able to climb out of it. Usually, that time has come when the side of the crib reaches the nipples of a standing child, although some clever children figure out how to make a getaway earlier than that. Remove large toys from the crib—the child can use them as stepping stones. The mattress should be at the lowest level and the crib sides raised at all times. Put a carpet or thick mat on the floor around the crib so that there will be a soft surface if (and when) the child does manage to climb out.

When it's time to forsake the crib, a small bed that is near ground level, a junior bed, is just fine. You can even use a mattress without a frame. But I wish parents wouldn't buy bunk beds. Even when there are rails on the top bunk, children manage to fall out. If you need to conserve space, a trundle-bed arrangement, whereby one bed slides under another, is safer.

NIGHTTIME INTERRUPTIONS

Everyone dreams of a newborn who sleeps through the night from the first day at home, and some parents are lucky enough to have such a baby. Most infants, however, take about three to four months to sleep through from bedtime to early morning. Even after they've established the habit of sleeping all night, about 20 percent of babies will abruptly start waking up again sometime in the first two years. This new pattern may last for several weeks. When I told one mother that this occurs in 1 out of 4 babies, she said, "Why do I only know the mothers of the other three?"

This sleep-wake pattern may be caused by a number of factors, including separation anxiety, hunger, and the teething process. Separation anxiety occurs normally from three to nine months, when a baby begins to realize that Mommy is a separate organism. If the baby awakens to find that Mommy is not there, the fear is that she may never return. With Mommy's reappearance, the child is generally reassured and will calm, often without cuddling or feeding. The parent who offers comfort at times of fear and anxiety is not being overindulgent. If you let the baby "cry it out," you'll only reinforce the child's fears of abandonment.

The most constructive response to a child who has awakened at night is to be there but to limit your interaction. If you can get by with just a peek into the room so that the child can see your face, that may be all that is needed. If the child wants to be held, do so for as short a time as possible, then gently put the child back down in the crib. The less stimulation and contact, the easier it will be for the child to fall back asleep and the less reinforcement there will be for the pattern to recur.

Hunger also causes babies to awaken at night. If your

baby still demands to be fed every two to four hours after the age of six months or more, the problem may be "trained night feeding." The baby's stomach is accustomed to being filled at those specific intervals, and the child awakens hungry even though there is no nutritional need for that extra feeding.

To wean your infant from nighttime feedings, gradually decrease the volume of each feeding. For babies who are formula-fed, decrease the volume by one-fourth of an ounce at each feeding. Such slight differences won't be noticed from one feeding to the next. If you're breast-feeding, time the feedings and gradually decrease each by fifteen to thirty seconds. The change will be insignificant from one feeding to the next, and the baby will no longer awaken hungry.

Babies accustomed to a feeding schedule of every three or four hours during the day are more likely to go longer at night. Avoid using the breast or bottle as a "comforter" during the day when the baby seems bored or fretful. It's all too easy for the child to demand the same kind of comfort during the night.

A substantial meal close to bedtime will not ensure a more prolonged sleep. It seems as though it should, but, for reasons no one understands, it doesn't. Food is not a means of keeping a child asleep.

Teething pain is another cause of wakefulness. Pain always feels more severe at night. If a baby over six months seems uncomfortable, try aspirin or acetaminophen (Tylenol, Panadol, Tempra, Liquiprin) according to the dosage schedule on page 154. If there's an obvious protrusion on the gums where a tooth is coming in, apply a topical teething gel such as Baby Orajel or Num·Zit directly to the swelling. See more about teething later in this chapter.

Some babies who have trouble staying asleep haven't

learned to fall back asleep by themselves. Both adults and children have a cyclical pattern of waking and sleeping through the night, and there are times when all of us reach a stage of slight awakening. Babies whose parents have talked to them or have picked them up every time they started to awaken or who need to have a pacifier to fall asleep again won't learn how to relax themselves back to sleep. The same may be true if parents allow a child to stay in their bedroom for too long. Your baby should not always require your presence to return to sleep.

Some babies remain wakeful if they are stimulated just before bedtime. This may be the only time working parents, especially fathers, have to spend with their children, and encouraging babies to coo and laugh is great fun. However, it's hard for them to settle down after such exciting activity. Most babies are better off with a quiet time before bed: rock the child in your arms, tell comforting stories, or sing gentle, quiet songs.

A mother once told me that her friend said it was time to give up rocking her three-year-old daughter to sleep. The mother said, "I love rocking my child to sleep for those ten minutes, and I always look forward to it." There's nothing wrong with giving your child that last little measure of comfort if this is what both of you want. Your child will grow up and out of those needs soon enough. If you hear advice to the contrary, smile, nod, and ignore it.

You'll see that I haven't recommended "crying it out." Childless people or those who have forgotten what it was like to have a baby may suggest this. But no matter how tired parents are, it's almost impossible for them not to respond to a child's desperate cries. Most parents who tell me that they tried to let a child cry it out have found that the strategy backfired. A baby can become severely upset and can throw up, or can become twisted in the bedclothes, and when this happens, the calming process will take longer.

It's not necessary to run to the crib every time your baby whimpers. Wait a few minutes, just long enough to see if the child will fall back asleep alone. A low, rhythmic noise in the room sometimes helps, such as a radio playing softly, the hum of a humidifier, a ticking clock, or one of the stuffed animals that has a recording inside simulating a heartbeat. Although you're relying temporarily on an artificial device, at least you will get some well-deserved sleep and your baby will eventually outgrow the need for your presence.

After all this, does it seem as though there's no single, simple answer to a sleep problem? Yes, but there are a few rules: don't respond at every whimper; try not to feed your baby through the night after the age of four to six months; and allow the baby to find his or her own way to return to sleep. If problems do arise, the solutions often have to be tailored to the particular situation. In a study conducted at Park Hospital in Oxford, England, families with sleep disorders each had different situations and distinct dynamics, attitudes, and priorities. The solutions were highly individual, and researchers were able to help each family only after a detailed investigation of what went on in each home. This parallels my own experience. Resolution of a continuing sleep problem may require further exploration with your pediatrician.

If the simple solutions I've outlined don't do the trick, you may have to consult your pediatrician. Meantime, if the problem isn't chronic, do what you feel is right. With common sense and love, you're not going to harm your child.

CRYING AND FUSSINESS

A baby cries not only because of hunger and pain but also to communicate feelings such as boredom, fear, and loneliness. Sometime between 5 P.M. and 10 P.M., for one to four hours, many babies have a fussy period when they cry inconsolably.

There is little you can do to alleviate the fretfulness. You walk, burp, change diapers, feed your child, and do anything else that comes to mind, but nothing seems to help. I call this the "unhappy hour." We all have biological rhythms, and many of us hit a low in the early evening, roughly from 5 P.M. to 7 P.M. Adults have a happy hour at the end of the day, when we run out of steam and relax. Babies seem to have a similar cycle. In the first few months, their days are very active and stimulating. By early evening, they've built up a lot of tension and fatigue. While grownups may unwind with a cocktail or a jog, a baby's primary release is to cry. Such fretful behavior usually ends by the time the child is six months old.

You might carry a fussing baby in a chest carrier while you proceed with your evening activities. If the baby is close to your heartbeat and body warmth, that may provide soothing security.

People often think that if crying ceases the moment a baby is picked up, this means the infant is spoiled. But think a minute. If your lover, spouse, or good friend were lonely and asked for your company, would you refuse it? We should certainly treat our children with the same warmth and closeness we would give our loved ones and friends. Spoiling is not a consideration here.

Infants quickly learn that mother feeds them and attends to bodily needs. Father then comes to mean "play" and a more social relationship. A father can often soothe the baby during a fussy period more easily than a mother, particularly one who has been on hand all day. As a new participant, a father serves an extremely important function.

COLIC

A colicky baby in your household is an unsettling experience for parents and a source of puzzlement for pediatricians. No one really knows what causes colic. It is manifested when an infant engages in high-pitched, prolonged screaming for no apparent reason. Some babies with colic seem to experience cramping abdominal pain because they draw their knees up and scream at intervals. Colic starts at about one month of age and stops by three or four months as abruptly as it began. Parents become fearful that there is something wrong with the child, and are often frustrated by their helplessness to alleviate the distress.

Babies do not develop colic because their parents aren't loving enough. It was once thought that colicky babies were the by-product of anxious mothers. Now we know that the mother's stress is more likely caused by the baby's colic rather than the other way around.

A small percentage of babies may be sensitive to a component of cow's milk. If you're breast feeding and drinking cow's milk, try eliminating it from your diet for a week or two. About one in five breast-feeding babies with colic will improve with this change alone. A bottle-fed baby receiving formula based on cow's milk, such as Enfamil, Similac, or SMA, might do better on a soy-based formula such as Isomil, Soyalac, or Neo-mull-Soy.

Movement can sometimes distract a baby from the discomfort of colic. Simply holding and rocking may help. You might try setting the infant stomach down on a hot water bottle or heating pad wrapped in a towel. But never use a heating pad directly on a child's sensitive skin. The movement of a waterbed mattress or windup swing may be soothing. Or you might put the child in an infant seat on top of the dishwasher or dryer for the gentle vibration of the running appliance. Keep a close watch if you do this, however, for the infant and seat could easily topple off.

Some babies are calmed by the sound of the vacuum cleaner. Just let it run. There are also devices on the market with the sounds of mother's heartbeat that may ease the crying. If all else fails, the motion of a car ride may do wonders for a fretful, colicky baby.

If there is a particularly disturbing crying period and nothing seems to help, try removing yourself from the situation for a little while. Step outside or take a shower, and renew your own energy and serenity.

Parents of all babies need some time away, and parents of babies with colic need it more than most. Don't feel guilty leaving your baby with another caretaker for a few hours. You will be a better parent if you can handle your infant with more equanimity.

Colic attacks may happen only during the day, if you're lucky, but are a frequent nighttime occurrence as well. If the simple measures I've suggested don't work, call your pediatrician. We know of no sure cure for colic, but prescription medications such as Donnatal or Levsin may relieve the symptoms.

It seems as though a child who has suffered so long and so acutely from colic should have difficulties later in life. However, there is no evidence of later problems. This is only one example of how infants and children are often tougher than we realize. When your baby is three or four months old and the attacks stop, just be relieved and catch up on some sleep yourself.

THUMBS AND PACIFIERS

Babies and toddlers need to suck even when they're not hungry because of the soothing nature of repetitive activity. We all need this at times. Adults may chew pencils, twirl their hair, or—less healthfully—overeat. Babies who are comforted by sucking aren't demonstrating insecurity, nor is this a reflection on the quality of parenting.

Some babies are even born with a sucking blister, a callouslike bump that develops on the thumb after prolonged, vigorous sucking. This is irrefutable evidence that they've been sucking their thumbs in the womb. I can't help but think that these babies have a head start in life, since they've already figured out how to comfort themselves.

Many people have the misconception that children should be prevented from thumb-sucking. The major reason given is that thumb-sucking may be responsible for crooked teeth later. People also seem to disapprove of the habit because they think it "looks bad" or they have the notion that a child beyond a certain age should be past the need for it.

In actual fact, thumb-sucking does not cause crooked or "buck" teeth, especially if the child stops the activity by the time the permanent teeth come through, as most children do. (The most severe thumb-sucking habit I've ever seen was in one of my seven-year-old patients. A Little League pitcher, he took his hand out of his glove to suck his thumb between pitches. This might have improved his game, but I hope he stops before he reaches the Majors. Incidentally, he doesn't have crooked teeth, even though he already has his permanent teeth.)

Some children prefer their thumbs, and others favor pacifiers. It's almost impossible to change a pacifier devotee to the thumb and vice versa. There's no reliable research about adverse effects of either pacifiers or thumbs, and most of what has been written or said is purely conjecture.

There are, however, pros and cons to both thumbs and pacifiers. Obviously, the thumb is always there. It can't be lost in bed like a pacifier. On the other hand, since it *is* always there, thumb-sucking may last longer than sucking on a pacifier.

As to types of pacifiers, so far as I can tell, there's no advantage to one kind over another. Some children like the shorter, orthodontically shaped ones, and others prefer the traditional nipple-shaped pacifiers. I don't think either type makes a difference in later orthodontic health. For obvious safety reasons, never attach a pacifier around a child's neck with a string or pin it to a toddler's clothes.

Most children will eventually confine their thumb-sucking to naptime and bedtime. There's no need to try to break the habit, and measures such as painting the thumb with bitter medicine only teach a child to tolerate the unpleasant taste. If the sight of a child sucking a thumb or pacifier bothers you, wait at least until the child is two or older to encourage him or her to give up the thumb. Even then, your efforts should only be positive: register approval when the child desists from thumb-sucking, but don't be disappointed if there are lapses. Above all, don't make a big deal out of this. The more you insist, the longer the child will hold onto the beloved habit.

TEETHING

When a baby about three months old becomes fussy, drools, and chews on everything within grasp, people say, "Oh, he's teething." Well, that could be true, and then again it may not be. Teething has been held responsible for fretfulness, diarrhea, fevers, drooling, and colds, not all of which are valid.

It's normal for babies to salivate more by the age of three or four months and to use their mouths to explore the world. During this period they chew on everything from keys to your favorite velvet cushion. Some children cut their first teeth at four months, but others may not have a single tooth until they're almost a year old. The rate and order in which teeth come in is enormously variable. The first teeth are usually the lower front incisors, but some babies acquire their upper teeth first, and some have eyeteeth before any others.

Some fortunate children have no problem with teething; suddenly a tooth is there. If teething is painful, baby aspirin or acetaminophen (see dosages, page 154) may alleviate the discomfort. If the tooth is visible, rub a little ice or an anesthetic teething gel such as Num·Zit or Baby Orajel on the gum. Be sparing with teething gels, however. The gel contains an anesthetic property and, if swallowed, can numb the throat, increasing the danger of choking.

At night, when you may not have access to a drugstore preparation, rub a little whiskey on the gum. The alcohol in the whiskey has an anesthetic effect.

Babies have to cut about twenty teeth in a year, and it's sometimes difficult to know whether a baby is really ill during this time or simply suffering from the discomfort of teething. As a general rule, if your baby has a fever of over 101 degrees Fahrenheit (or 38 degrees Centigrade) or is fretful for more than one day, consult your doctor. An ear infection or some other problem may be the cause of the discomfort.

As teeth break through the gums, there may be an "eruption cyst," a swelling on the gum that looks like a blood-filled bruise. It looks, and probably is, painful. There is no need to lance the cyst or use anything other than the pain-relieving tactics I've already mentioned. In a day or two, when the tooth erupts, the swelling will disappear.

Is there a relationship between teething and other illnesses? Many children contract colds or have diarrhea when they begin to teethe. When the gums are stimulated in the teething process, the stomach may think that food is on the way, and the entire gastrointestinal tract may increase its activity. This can sometimes cause loose stools. If your child has persistent diarrhea for more than a day, it's probably caused by something other than teething.

Runny noses seem to accompany teething, but teeth begin to erupt at the same time children start catching colds. As far as I know, there is no medical connection between colds and the developmental process of teething, nor can tooth eruption cause a significant fever.

Start cleaning a child's teeth as soon as they appear. Dentists recommend brushing after every meal, but infants and children eat so frequently that you'd spend half your day cleaning teeth. When your child has two or more teeth, use a soft baby toothbrush, a piece of gauze wrapped around your finger, or a soft terry washcloth, with or without toothpaste. Gently wipe all surfaces of the teeth. Do this at least three times a day, especially before naps and bedtime. When children are ready to brush their teeth themselves, make sure you do a follow-up, since an eighteen- or twenty-four-month-old child cannot be relied on to do an adequate job.

Dentists recommend that children have their first dental

visit at age three unless there are problems that require attention earlier. That earlier attention can be avoided if you start preventive care as soon as the teeth appear.

MINOR MEDICAL CONDITIONS IN THE FIRST WEEKS

Newborn Acne

Nearly 40 percent of babies develop infant acne or newborn acne at the end of the first month. Some have only a mild case; in others, it's more severe. Acne is a rash that first appears on the face and may extend to the shoulders and scalp. It consists of little pus-filled pimples on a red base. The rash is more conspicuous at some times than others, but it doesn't disappear until the infant is two or three months old. Acne is not related to heat rash, although it seems to become worse when the baby is warm.

No one knows what causes infant acne, nor does anyone know whether babies with infant acne are destined to have later acne. The only sure thing is that the rash always seems to grow worse just before you want to take your baby's picture or when your out-of-town relatives come to visit.

There's nothing you can do to shorten the course of acne. Just wash the baby's face with clear water, and the situation will resolve itself in a month or two.

Cradle Cap

Cradle cap, or seborrhea, is an infant form of dandruff. It's seen often in infants and is more obvious in babies with thin or light hair. There may be a slight scaliness to the scalp, or there can be patches of thick, greasy brownish scales adhering to the scalp.

The treatment of cradle cap involves removing the scales and preventing their return. To loosen them, apply warm olive oil or baby oil to the scalp half an hour before shampooing. The scales may become transparent, but they're still there. Then wash with a gentle dandruff shampoo such as Sebulex or Head & Shoulders, using a soft baby toothbrush or hairbrush, scrubbing the scaly area rather briskly. Of course, avoid getting dandruff shampoo in the baby's eyes.

Don't hesitate to scrub vigorously over the baby's soft spot (the diamond-shaped depression on the top of the head). There's a tough membrane beneath this depression, between the brain and the skin, and you won't do any harm by rubbing the scalp in this area. Although the area is usually slightly depressed, it may bulge a bit when the baby cries. That's normal.

If cradle cap doesn't respond to these simple measures or if the rash extends to other areas, your doctor may prescribe a mild cortisone cream.

Blocked Tear Duct

The tear duct is that small opening on the inside corner of the lower eyelid. A constant stream of tears washes across our eyes to lubricate them and to remove impurities, and the fluid drains through the duct into the nose. That's why we have to blow our nose when we cry.

In most newborns this duct is open, but in some infants who haven't developed an open tear duct you can see a constant puddle of tears in the lower part of the baby's eye. These excess tears may occasionally spill over even when the baby is not crying, and there may be some white or yellow mucus occasionally at the inner corner of the eye.

An obstructed tear duct will usually open by the time a child is one year old. If this hasn't happened, a simple surgical procedure performed by an ophthalmologist may be necessary. Before that time, some pediatricians advise parents to massage the inner corner of the eye several times a day. If there is mucus or pus draining from the eye, antibiotic eye drops may be prescribed. No one knows if massage actually helps. I think that these ducts probably open when they are destined to open, and all the massage and drops in the world won't make them open earlier.

EIGHT

Illness: What Did I Do Wrong?

MY HUSBAND thinks I should have a blackboard in my waiting room listing specials of the day, much as restaurants do. On my blackboard he suggests I write "Malade du jour" or "What's going around." Although any "going-around disease" certainly causes distress and sick children, parents seem reassured when I tell them that half the neighborhood has the same infection.

Some babies and children catch whatever is going around, and others never seem to be laid low. Yet all children, whether sick or well, are constantly warding off infection and producing antibodies that help prevent more serious illness in adulthood. Before the advent of mumps vaccine, 30 percent of people who were found to have antibodies to mumps in their bloodstream had no history of mumps disease. They had the infection nonetheless, and their bodies manufactured antibodies to it. The same is true for myriad other illnesses.

Each child has a particular way of responding to illness. In children with a tendency toward allergies, the membranes of the respiratory tract swell and fill with mucus, making them a good host for germs. Other children seem to vomit whenever they're ill, and still others run a high fever with each infection. As your child grows and develops, there probably will be a series of minor illnesses. This should be no cause for worry; he or she is developing normally, catching and fighting infections.

Any sickness is more severe at night, and that's not just your imagination. Although primitive peoples believed that evil spirits were abroad in the dark, the truth of the matter is that fevers are elevated at night because of our normal daily temperature cycle, which is lowest early in the morning and highest late at night. Illness does seem more frightening at three in the morning than in the light of day. We have fewer people around to help, our wits are not as sharp, and children as well as adults focus on their discomfort simply because other distractions are not available. Pediatricians are quite accustomed to nocturnal phone calls from concerned parents.

Sometimes parents call me at night because their child has a high fever or a cough or ear pain, and then they arrive at the office or emergency room with a child who is alert and playful, full of vim and vigor. The child who wouldn't take fluids is sucking happily on a bottle; the child who couldn't breathe without coughing is singing and cooing. At that point parents are torn between relief and embarrassment, insisting, "But he really looked terrible at home—really!"

Don't be embarrassed if this happens to you. I've thought of bottling a medication called Elixir of Trip to the Office (the industrial strength would be Elixir of Trip to the Emergency Room) since so many problems resolve themselves spontaneously once help seems assured. The ear still needs to be checked, the chest to be listened to, but somehow the acute stage of the problem has subsided.

I find myself continually telling parents that they are not to blame for a child's illness. Only in old movies do going without a sweater and becoming chilled lead to pneumonia; putting on a hat does not keep a child from getting an ear infection. There is no disease or infection I can imagine for which parents can blame themselves unless they want to feel guilty for their genetic predispositions. For example, parents who suffered from allergies as children may have children whose allergic tendencies make them more susceptible to minor infections.

One of the many nice things about taking care of children is that they get well very quickly and they really *want* to be well. They'll jump out of bed and play as soon as they feel better; but they will also, unlike adults, go willingly to bed if they're not well. As adults, we often push ourselves beyond good sense, but children never do that.

Formerly, children with rheumatic fever were confined to bed for six weeks. In one of the hospitals where I trained, pedometers, devices that measure movement, were attached to the ankles and wrists of children with rheumatic fever. One group of children was allowed to be up and playing quietly; the other group remained in bed. It was discovered that the children who were confined to bed after they felt well enough to play measured more activity on the pedometer than the group that was allowed to play. In other words, a child who feels well will become restless and more active. The child should be allowed to set the limits for activity according to how he or she feels. Trying to confine a child who doesn't feel like being in bed is futile and counterproductive.

In this chapter, I will discuss the common illnesses children face in the first two years. This is by no means a comprehensive treatment of all the possible medical problems any child can face, but I will cover the infections and medical problems that I see in the office and about which I talk to parents most often.

FEVER

What constitutes a fever? Normal body temperature is 98.6 degrees Fahrenheit or 36.5 degrees Centigrade, but that is only an average. While normal body temperature can range from 97 to 99.5 at rest, activity and a high ambient temperature can elevate it. An active child can have a body temperature of 101 degrees Fahrenheit simply because he or she is active, and a child playing outdoors on a very hot day may also register a fever.

Fevers are caused by a chemical released by our white blood cells as they mobilize our defenses against infection. Such a universal phenomenon must have some function, some adaptive value. Lizards, which depend on outside sources for their body heat, deliberately raise their body temperatures when they contract infection. If denied access to a heat source, the lizard will succumb to the infection. In other words, lizards need fever to fight infection, and the same is probably true of humans.

What this implies is that fever has a value and in and of itself should not be treated. Yet fevers make children and adults uncomfortable with headaches and body pain and general misery, and sometimes we need to treat fever simply to relieve discomfort.

Doctors consider a temperature over 101 degrees Fahrenheit in an infant or child and over 100 degrees Fahrenheit in a newborn up to age one month to be in the fever range. Sometimes children just feel warm, but their temperature is normal; a child's skin may warm up before body temperature has risen because the body is trying to lose some of the heat being generated. A little later the thermometer may reflect the rise in body temperature.

Temperatures should always be taken when a child has been at rest. A temperature taken rectally is most accurate, but you must be very careful inserting the thermometer, not an easy task if a baby is wiggling. There is always the risk of damaging tissue, so I usually advise against taking a temperature rectally in infants and small children. Axillary (or armpit) temperatures are less accurate but are easier and safer. The thermometer should rest directly on the skin. Keep the child's arm firmly against the thermometer for three to five minutes. You can obtain an accurate reading if you sit in a rocking chair and hug the child tightly for that three-to-five-minute period. An oral reading is safe and fairly accurate, but infants and small children have difficulty holding the thermometer under their tongues with their mouths closed.

Fever strips, which are placed against a child's forehead and which register a chemically induced color change, are inaccurate. Yet they may be better than nothing if you have difficulty reading a thermometer (and a surprising number of people do). The strips can at least indicate that the child has a fever, although not the degree of fever.

Strict accuracy as to a child's temperature is not all that important. You only need to have an approximate reading and to know whether the temperature is rising or falling. The difference between, say, a temperature of 101.2 degrees Fahrenheit and 101.8 degrees Fahrenheit is not critical.

Many people think they should add a degree or two to an axillary temperature reading because the degree registered is lower than with a rectal thermometer. When reporting to your doctor, give the temperature reading and the manner in which it was obtained, and use the same technique for further readings. The difference in temperature readings between axillary and rectal methods is not uniform, and converting values is not necessary or reliable.

If you don't trust your reading of a thermometer, your lips and hands are still a reasonably accurate gauge. A baby who is flushed, whose skin feels as though you could fry an egg on it, has a high fever. If the baby's skin is warmer than yours but not hot, the fever is mild, and that's useful information for the doctor. With experience, many mothers can tell by feel what temperature a child has within a degree.

Your child may look or act sick before you even detect a fever. Since activity raises body temperature, a feverish child's first response may be to go to bed or lie listlessly in your arms or in a crib. This natural response keeps the body from generating more heat. In order to lose some of the excess heat, the blood vessels near the surface of the skin enlarge, to expose more blood to the cooler air. This makes a child look flushed and feverish.

When body temperature rises, the heart rate increases and becomes stronger. Children's chests are not padded with breast tissue and lots of muscle, and so when parents hold a feverish child, they often feel the child's heart pounding. This is only because of the fever, and the heart rate will return to normal as the fever subsides, with no subsequent damage to the child's heart. Your child may breathe a little faster with a fever, but this will also subside when the fever goes down. If a child is having no difficulty breathing, there's nothing wrong with the lungs.

The degree of fever is not a criterion as to whether or not a child needs medication or fever-fighting attention. Rather, judge by how the child seems to be feeling. A temperature of 99 or 100 degrees Fahrenheit certainly doesn't call for medication, but if a child is uncomfortable, a little acetaminophen (Tylenol, Panedol, Tempra) may help. Conversely, a temperature of 103 degrees Fahrenheit, while upsetting to parents when they read the thermometer, doesn't require treatment if the child seems otherwise comfortable. Pathologically high temperatures occur only in special circumstances, such as with heat stroke or after prolonged exposure to the hot sun.

If the fever is high and your child seems uncomfortable, remove all clothing except the diaper to help the body exchange heat with the air. The theory that people with fevers should "sweat it out" arose because when a fever breaks a person may perspire. Hindsight, then, has it that if you cause sweating you'll break a fever.

Sponging the head and shoulders with lukewarm water cools the skin surface. If the child starts to shiver, stop sponging and replace the clothes or wrap the child in a blanket. Shivering is the body's mechanism for generating heat and means that cooling is too rapid. Be sure not to use cold water for sponging: think of how it would feel to be plunged in a tub of cold water, even if you didn't have a fever. Babies, shocked by cold water, will scream, and prolonged screaming itself can raise body temperature.

There's another, more important reason to use only tepid water. When any part of the body has been chilled, the natural response is for blood vessels at the surface of the skin to constrict. Therefore, cold water may even raise the fever, for the skin cannot lose heat if the blood vessels cannot dilate. Cold water was at one time the general policy in emergency rooms. Nurses would call me because they were trying to cool a feverish child and instead the temperature was rising. When I would instruct them to stop the cold treatment, the fever would subside. Fortunately, most emergency-room doctors and nurses have stopped trying to use ice to reduce fever.

Water used for sponging should be at body temperature —barely warm on your wrist. For many years people have used alcohol because it seems to cool the skin more quickly. However, fumes from evaporating alcohol can make both baby and parent feel sick. Water does the job just as well and doesn't have any side effects.

I've left the discussion of fever medications for last because medicine should not be your first response. Often, the simple measures of removing clothes and sponging the child's head and shoulders will bring down a fever. However, if a child is still uncomfortable, there are two drugs that may be used: aspirin and acetaminophen.

Aspirin, which has been around for a long time, is very effective, but, as with any effective medication, it also has side effects. A high level of aspirin in the blood can be toxic, and a feverish child who's not taking fluids well and may be somewhat dehydrated, has greater susceptibility to toxic blood levels. Aspirin can cause allergic reactions and may have a direct effect on the airway resistance of children with asthma, causing them to wheeze more. Aspirin also affects the mechanism of blood clotting and irritates the lining of the stomach.

There have been reports of the possible association of aspirin and Reye's syndrome, a very rare but serious and potentially fatal liver problem of unknown cause that occurs in children after certain viral infections, especially chickenpox and influenza. Since the public-information campaign to warn parents of this potential danger, the incidence of Reye's syndrome in children has declined significantly.

If aspirin were newly developed today, it probably would not be approved by the FDA, and certainly would not be available without a prescription. However, aspirin in appropriate doses to treat a simple fever not associated with chickenpox or flu is probably safe. Acetaminophen, however, is a safer drug. It comes under various trade names such as Tylenol, Tempra, Panedol, and Liquiprin. There are fewer allergic reactions to acetaminophen than to aspirin, and its toxicity in children is low compared to aspirin. Also, acetaminophen comes in a liquid preparation, whereas children's aspirin comes in the form of a chewable tablet, not appropriate for babies and toddlers.

Both acetaminophen and aspirin should be administered no more than every four hours. For a recalcitrant high fever and a child who is in obvious discomfort, you might alternate acetaminophen and aspirin every three hours. Remember that we're treating something that's an appropriate bodily response to infection, and we shouldn't risk drug toxicity simply to lower a fever.

A final word of caution: any temperature over 100 degrees Fahrenheit in an infant under one month should be reported immediately to your pediatrician. Fevers in newborns are of greater concern since immunity is not well developed. Even a slight fever may indicate a serious infection. After the first month, you don't have to worry about every fever. Use your judgment and consider not only the degree of the fever but how the child looks. If your child isn't acting sick, you might wait a day to see what develops.

DOSAGES TO TREAT FEVER

	2 to 6 months	6 to 12 months	1 to 2 years
Acetaminophen drops	.3 or .4 ml.	.6 or .8 ml.	1.2 or 1.6 ml.
Acetaminophen elixir		½ tsp.	¾ to 1 tsp.
Chewable tablets			1 tab.

To summarize, here are the steps to take if your child has a fever:

1. Remove excess clothing, and dress the child in light pajamas or a diaper.
2. Sponge the child's head and shoulders with lukewarm water, or put the baby in a tepid bath, but stop sponging if you observe shivering.
3. Use an appropriate dose of acetaminophen or aspirin.
4. If your baby is less than one month old or looks sick even if the fever is not high, call the pediatrician.
5. If the fever persists for longer than twenty-four hours, call the doctor.
6. Don't use alcohol or cold water to bathe the baby.
7. Don't panic. Remember that fever itself is not harmful.

Fever Convulsions

About one in twenty children under five years of age have fever convulsions. Children may shake, roll their eyes up, become limp or stiff, then look dazed or sleepy. They will recover completely, acting perfectly normal a few minutes later. Generally, a febrile seizure lasts no longer than five minutes, though it can seem an hour to worried parents.

Some doctors think that the important factor in precipitating a seizure is not how high the temperature becomes but rather the rate at which it rises. We're not sure about the cause, but we do know that having a febrile seizure does not mean that your child has or will have epilepsy. Anyone whose child has had a febrile seizure wants to be sure that it never happens again, but, unfortunately, there isn't a lot you can do about that. The overwhelming majority of children have only one episode, but a few children experience more than one. You can't prevent your child from getting a fever, and you certainly can't control the rate at which it rises.

With a fever convulsion, a child for a short while may turn blue from holding his or her breath at the onset of the seizure. There are several protective measures you can take. Turn the child's head to the side so that saliva or food will drain from the mouth. Don't use your finger or any other implement to keep the child from "swallowing his or her tongue." This doesn't happen, and clumsy attempts to insert something in the mouth can be harmful.

Sponge the child with lukewarm water, and wait for the seizure to be over. If you've had CPR (cardiopulmonary resuscitation) training (and everyone should have it), you will know how to insure that the child's airway is clear. If you don't know how to do this and are frightened, call the paramedics at 911 or your local emergency number and ask for instructions. After the seizure has run its course, call your pediatrician and describe what happened and how the child is behaving now.

Pediatricians often have to deal with fever seizures, and constantly reassure parents that the seizures are not serious. However, not even pediatricians can be level-headed when their own children are involved. One of my colleagues brought his child into the emergency room, wrapped in a wet towel. In a panic, he threw the child into my lap, saying, "Save him, save him!" When your own offspring is having a seizure, it's difficult to be cool and rational. If you read this before your child has such a convulsion, it may help you.

Medicine to prevent seizures, when given by mouth, takes twenty-four to forty-eight hours to reach effective blood levels, at which point a child's fever has usually subsided. To prevent febrile seizures, you would have to administer medication every day for years. It's hardly justifiable to administer a drug with multiple side effects for something that is not life-threatening and that is unlikely to recur.

Roseola

While febrile convulsions may be asociated with many infections, roseola (infant measles) is the most common. Roseola affects children from the ages of six months to nineteen months. It drives pediatricians nuts because children run an erratic high fever for three to five days and there are no other symptoms or physical findings. It's the only disease I know of where a rash appears *after* the fever is gone. The diagnosis can only be made after the rash appears, but in the meantime parents and pediatricians keep watching the child closely because they're never absolutely certain until they see the rash.

The rash—light pink and in scattered spots all over the body, including the face—does not itch. It disappears without complications in one or two days.

Antibiotics are not necessary or effective in treating infant measles. Simply keep the child as comfortable as possible following the measures outlined under fever on page 154, and make sure there is good fluid intake even if the baby has no appetite for food.

RESPIRATORY INFECTIONS

Colds

All that sniffles is not a cold. A stuffy or runny nose can result from allergy or irritation due to smog, smoke, or dry indoor air. A cold is a viral infection that causes a runny nose, usually with clear mucus, and sometimes a cough and a slight fever. Babies can't clear their throats or sniff, so whatever mucus they develop in their nose and throat makes them sound congested, although they may be happily eating and sleeping. A cold usually makes a child sick and uncomfortable.

Babies with colds have all the miseries adults have—they're fretful, cough, sneeze, have a meager appetite, and sleep poorly. Everybody knows there's no cure for a cold. Nevertheless, parents often bring children with colds to us on the mistaken notion that if we "catch it early," we can keep it from becoming worse.

As long as the mucus is clear or milky white, there's little to do and little we need do. My cousin Tyler had a runny nose for the first nine months of his life, and my dear Auntie Beenie was convinced that if I were his pediatrician, I would have had this condition cleared up in no time. It was hard to convince her that I wouldn't have done any better than his own pediatrician. The runny nose would have cleared up in its own time no matter who was taking care of him.

Mucus draining from the nose may be clear, white, yellow, or green. If your child has a yellow, foul-smelling discharge from only one nostril, however, that almost always means that the child has inserted something into it that shouldn't be there. Over the years, I've removed small stones, nuts, and other foreign objects from the nostrils of children between the ages of one and five.

Parents feel responsible when their small children come down with colds, but there's no way to prevent your child from contracting a cold or other infection and still live a normal life. Studies have shown that vitamin C has no consistent positive effect on colds. At the University of Sydney, in the study I find most convincing, researchers enrolled ninety-five pairs of identical twins. One of each set of twins received vitamin C and the other a placebo, and the frequency, duration, and intensity of colds were noted. According to the results, vitamin C had no effect on the incidence, total number, and average severity or intensity of the colds. In some cases, it did shorten the duration of a cold. Therefore, my feeling is that vitamin C doesn't help very much.

As with all viral infections, colds are not sensitive to antibiotics. So any self-respecting doctor will prescribe antibiotics for a child with a cold only if there are specific complications such as ear infection.

The purpose of cold medicines is to reduce discomfort, and these medications are available with or without a prescription in a variety of preparations. The ones that require a prescription are no stronger or more effective than the others, but they *are* more expensive. In my opinion, none of them is worth recommending, and they're not without negative effects. For example, decongestants can make children nervous and sleepless, irritable and even more uncomfortable than they already are. Decongestants can also cause hallucinations in children, which cause no permanent damage but can frighten children and parents unnecessarily.

There are some things parents can do to alleviate cold symptoms. The most obvious way to unplug a nose would seem to be nose drops with virtually instant results, but nothing is that simple. With small babies, nose drops are absorbed into the bloodstream and can cause side-effects. Also, with frequent use nose drops cause a rebound phenomenon—the more often you use them, the more dependent you become on them.

Nevertheless, nose drops are effective and safe when used in a limited way. Use them only at times of extreme discomfort when the child can't get to sleep or drink a bottle, and never for more than two or three days. Use one drop in each nostril at bedtime or just before a feeding once or twice a day at most.

Moisturizing the air in a child's room may make the child more comfortable. For safety reasons I recommend a humidifier, which creates a fine, cool mist, rather than a vaporizer, which turns water into steam.

An infant with a stuffed nose and mucus draining into the throat will also sleep more comfortably with the head elevated. You can raise the crib mattress on one end or have the baby sleep in an infant seat.

Some people think that infants and children shouldn't drink milk or formula because it is mucus-forming, but this isn't true. It may be easier, however, for a small baby to suck clear liquids through a nipple when the nose is blocked.

It takes about a week to ten days for a cold to run its course no matter what you do. Children may have a residual cough or running nose for two or three weeks thereafter. But if the condition is mild, doesn't disturb sleep, and isn't associated with fever, there's no need for any treatment.

Ear Infections

An infant who has a middle-ear infection, known medically as otitis media, will cry, hold the ear, or dig into an ear with a finger. There may or may not be a fever, and occasionally yellowish matter will drain from the ear.

While an infected ear may not cause pain, most children have some discomfort and have various degrees of irritability ranging from crankiness to prolonged screaming. Acetaminophen (Tylenol, Tempra, Panadol, and so forth) or aspirin can be effective pain relievers. The dosage is as follows:

DOSAGE TO TREAT EAR INFECTIONS

	2 to 6 months	6 to 12 months	1 to 2 years
Acetaminophen drops	.3 or .4 ml.	.6 or .8 ml.	1.2 or 1.6 ml.
Acetaminophen elixir		½ tsp.	¾ to 1 tsp.
Chewable tablets			1 tab.

These medications will be effective within the hour. For more immediate relief, warm a small amount of oil—mineral, olive, or salad—and fill the ear canal using an eye dropper. Infants up to one year need only one or two drops, older children may need four or five. If the ear is draining, do not administer the oil. Until you can see your pediatrician, apply a hot water bottle to the sore ear. Even a simple measure such as hugging your child against your warm chest may bring some quick relief.

Whenever the possibility of ear infection exists, the child should be examined by a pediatrician. Earaches are not always due to ear infections. I've seen supposed ear infections that were anything from a foreign body in the ear to a strep throat with pain referred to the ear area.

A significant percentage of ear infections can lead to complications such as mastoid infections. Therefore, pediatricians treat all ear infections with a ten-day course of antibiotics, which also shorten the course of fever and alleviate pain. Antibiotics are usually effective within twenty-four to forty-eight hours, although some children seem to improve dramatically after only one dose.

For immediate pain relief, your doctor can prescribe ear drops that contain a topical anesthetic. This is one of the few prescriptions you should keep on hand even after the infection has resolved. Ear infections have a way of recurring. In fact, some of my colleagues present their patients with a prescription for these drops in the first weeks of a baby's life so that babies can receive prompt relief if they need it.

Even with faithful administration of medication, 10 to 15 percent of ear infections will not clear up with one course of medication. I always recheck the ear and have children return when they have finished their medication. If there is still fluid or inflammation in the middle ear, I try another antibiotic.

Since ear infections are so common, children may have several each year. Unfortunately, covering a child's ear in the wind or avoiding water in the ears at bathtime will not lessen the frequency of ear infections. An open passage called the Eustachian tube, whose function is to equalize pressure, runs from the back of the throat to the middle ear. In babies and young children, the Eustachian tube is short and narrow, and becomes occluded easily if the tissues in the area swell because of a cold or allergy. The only outside factor that may make a difference in the frequency of ear infections is the way in which the child drinks from a bottle. If the child is lying flat, milk flows past the opening to the Eustachian tube and can cause irritation and swelling, leading to repeated infections. Babies should either be propped on a pillow, be set in an infant seat, or, ideally, be held in a parent's arms while drinking from a bottle.

The most important factor with regard to the long-term consequences of recurring otitis is whether or not the ears heal completely between episodes. If your pediatrician sees a normal eardrum and your child can hear normally, there will be no problem despite recurring ear infections. Occasionally a referral to an ear, nose, and throat doctor may be necessary to evaluate whether there is persistent fluid in the middle ear. In that case, a minor surgical procedure might be indicated to equalize pressure in the middle ear and prevent further infections.

Sore Throat, Strep Throat, Tonsillitis, and Scarlet Fever

Infants with sore throats usually have a fever, and may refuse to eat or drink, may swallow with difficulty, or may stick fingers deep into their mouths. A sore throat can be caused by strep bacteria or a virus.

If a child has a fever, an inflamed throat, and swollen glands in the neck, we take a throat culture to see if this is a streptococcal infection. The back of the throat and tonsils are swabbed, and in twenty-four hours strep germs will grow on a culture plate. If no strep germs are present, the throat culture will be reported as "negative for strep."

Children whose throat cultures are negative for strep probably have a viral sore throat. These don't respond to antibiotics and generally resolve themselves in a few days. In the meantime, a parent can give the child acetaminophen (Tylenol, Panadol, Tempra, and so forth) for pain and fever, and can make sure there is adequate fluid intake, administering water or juice (Popsicles are also good—they have a cooling effect and distract the child).

If the culture is positive for strep, the child should receive a ten-day course of antibiotics or, in some cases, a single injection of penicillin. Years ago, rheumatic fever was not infrequently a well-recognized complication of strep infection. This is rare today, but we treat strep infections promptly with antibiotics in order to hasten recovery and to prevent spreading the infection to other children. Children with strep throats are contagious until they've received two days of antibiotics.

Scarlet fever is a strep infection accompanied by a rash. The disease begins with a fever and sore throat; on the second or third day of illness a rash of tiny red bumps appear in the armpits and groin. As the rash spreads to the rest of the body, the spots merge, leaving the skin feeling rough and sandpapery. The tongue develops a white coating, which then sloughs off, leaving a smooth, red surface with scattered bumps, which is called a "strawberry tongue." In some cases the skin may peel from the palms of the hands and the soles of the feet ten to fourteen days after the rash appears. Because of the possibility of contagion, children with scarlet fever should be isolated from other children for the first forty-eight hours of medication. We treat scarlet fever as we do a strep throat—with ten days of antibiotic.

Tonsillitis is not a separate infection, the term refers to an inflammation of the tonsils that accompanies a sore throat, whether of viral or bacterial origin.

Coughs

When a child coughs, the body is attempting to expel material, either real or imagined, from the airway. Sometimes, there really is mucus or pus in the air tubes, in which case there will be a moist-sounding, "productive" cough. Other times, however, the membranes lining the airways are irritated because of a cold or an allergic reaction, and the lungs are triggered to cough even though there is nothing to expel. This common type of dry cough occurs most often with a cold and may persist for days or weeks after the cold has disappeared. In general, these coughs are more severe when the child is lying down or is playing actively and is out of breath.

When a child with a cold is coughing, decongestants usually don't help. A humidifier in the child's bedroom at night may help to alleviate symptoms, and over-the-counter cough medicines with dextromethorphan (DM on the label) may help all of you to get much needed rest. If the cough is persistent, your pediatrician may prescribe medication with codeine for a night or two. For a child over one year who is coughing at night, try a mixture of one or two teaspoons of whiskey, a little honey, and lemon juice. This mixture generally helps parents to relax, too, if they take it themselves.

Another type of cough may be related to croup. Croup is a distinctive hollow cough that starts suddenly at night, often after a day or two of cold symptoms. The cough, which resembles a seal in distress, comes in paroxysms and is painful to a child's throat.

High humidity helps to alleviate symptoms. By running a hot shower with the bathroom doors and windows closed, you can create a steam-bath effect. You can also create a mist tent in the child's room by placing a humidifier on a chair next to the crib and draping a fabric sheet (*never* plastic) over both the crib and chair to concentrate the mist. The child's pajamas will become damp and should be changed often.

Cough medicines don't relieve croup, but a car ride in the night air (believe it or not) is one of the most effective treatments. Pediatricians understand this strategy through experience—it's not usually taught in medical school. Hearing the distressing coughs in the background when a parent calls, the pediatrician says, "Bring that child to the emergency room," expecting to see a very sick child. What the pediatrician often encounters is a calm baby with no symptoms of croup. The relaxing ride has worked its magic and has temporarily solved the problem.

If a ride in the night air doesn't help, an inhalation treatment may be administered at the hospital emergency room. A few drops of medication mixed with a salt solution and administered in a nebulized mist usually provides significant relief.

Allergies, especially asthma, can also be a cause of coughing. Asthma is characterized by wheezing, a high-pitched sound made when the breath is expelled. The wheezing is often apparent to the naked ear, but sometimes asthma can't be diagnosed until a pediatrician listens with a stethoscope. The spaces between the ribs may retract when the child breathes in, causing the ribs to look prominent. Breathing is apt to be rapid and shallow. In childhood asthma, there is often a family history of allergies.

The type of asthma medications prescribed will vary according to the preference of your pediatrician and the child's age. Most often treatment will involve administration of bronchodilators (to relax the airways) in liquid form. The prescription may be for Somophyllin, Theo-Dur, Slo-bid, Alupent, or Metaprel, to name a few possibilities. If your child is experiencing significant respiratory distress, your doctor or the emergency-room physician may try an injection of epinephrine (adrenaline). When effective, it will provide almost instantaneous relief.

One episode of wheezing does not constitute asthma. Wheezing can be associated with other conditions, such as the viral infection bronchiolitis. This is most common in infants from six to eighteen months and causes inflammation and spasms of the small airways, which is accompanied by a sound that resembles the wheezing of asthma.

The medications that are useful for asthma may also be effective for bronchiolitis. Since the side effects of these medications seem to be exaggerated in infants, we prescribe them sparingly. The medications can cause irritability and upset stomachs, and while they may relieve the wheezing, the baby may be fretting and wakeful.

Although minor viral infections lead to residual coughs that may last from four to six weeks, a severe cough or one that persists longer than a month should be called to your pediatrician's attention. Sometimes a chronic cough is not the result of an infection. A persistent cough may indicate that a small foreign body has lodged in the child's lungs. I've seen an array of material removed from children's lungs, including the foot of a Snoopy doll, a small weed, and an antique Yugoslavian coin. X-rays can usually identify the presence of a foreign body, and most objects can be removed with a special instrument while the child is lightly anesthetized.

Pneumonia

Parents have an understandable apprehension about a diagnosis of pneumonia, but most cases of pneumonia in children are not serious and certainly not life-threatening. They result from a viral respiratory infection accompanied by fever and cough. Pneumonia is an infection of the tissues of the lung. Your doctor may diagnose pneumonia simply by listening to the child's chest or may confirm the initial diagnosis with an x-ray.

If the cause is viral, pnuemonia won't respond to antibiotics, just as a cold or viral infection won't respond to antibiotics. Some cases of pneumonia are caused by bacteria. The children who contract this type of pneumonia may be somewhat sicker than those who have a viral pneumonia, with a high fever and more severe cough. It's frequently difficult to distinguish viral from bacterial pneumonia, so pediatricians treat most cases with antibiotics. With bacterial pneumonia, you will usually see a dramatic resolution of fever and other symptoms within twenty-four to forty-eight hours after antibiotics are begun.

Coughing doesn't always accompany pneumonia. A few years ago I saw a little boy in my office on a Friday afternoon. Justin was alert and his usual adorable self, except for a high fever. When his physical examination and urinalysis were normal, I suggested that his mother and I assume he had a viral infection and keep in close contact to see what developed. Two days later, on Sunday, since he still had a fever, I met them in the emergency room, where Justin was running around happily in his diaper, eating a graham cracker, and charming the staff. I looked over him with a fine-toothed comb and still couldn't find anything. His mother, who was an x-ray technician, said, "I think he has pneumonia." I told her I couldn't hear anything in his chest, but she said she couldn't help thinking he had it anyway. I asked if she'd feel better if we took a chest x-ray, all the time thinking that I was doing it just to humor her.

You guessed it. There on the x-ray was a large, probably bacterial pneumonia in the right upper lobe. This was a demonstration to me once again that mothers know their children better than pediatricians ever will. It also proved that pneumonia can be very clever at disguising itself.

After twenty-four hours of antibiotics, Justin's fever disappeared and a week later his chest x-ray was clear. This is the usual pattern of recovery in children, although they may take a few more days to return to normal.

Most pneumonias are contagious, and children should avoid contact with others until the fever has subsided and the cough diminishes. This will usually take two to five days.

GIVING CHILDREN MEDICATION

Liquid medication for children is usually prescribed by the teaspoon or half teaspoon. Your own silver teaspoon is not an accurate measure. The only reliable way to dispense liquid medicine is with a measuring spoon or a special dispensing spoon that can be purchased at your local drug store.

Don't mix a measured dose of medicine with formula or other liquids. If the baby doesn't finish the entire bottle, you won't know how much of the medicine has been ingested.

Read the directions on a bottle of medicine carefully each time you administer it. You may think that you remember the instructions from last time, but mistakes are often made. I once prescribed some *oral* drops for a baby with a cold, and his mother (who happened to be the wife of an ear, nose, and throat doctor) realized afterward that she had put the drops in the baby's nose. The medication didn't do any good, but fortunately, in this case, no harm was done either. However, memory is unreliable, particularly if you are anxious. Avoid mistakes by rereading directions.

Most people forget to give at least a few doses of medication; only about 20 percent of patients take all medicine as prescribed. Once an illness is over, many people save the remaining medication for "the next time." Don't do this. Your pediatrician would rather have you call in the middle of the night and prescribe new medication than have you decide when and how to medicate. While little or no harm may result from "leftovers," there is always the possibility that a former medication may be inappropriate or even obscure an important diagnosis. Also, your pediatrician may have more effective measures to suggest when a problem occurs.

"Isn't there a shot you can give him?" is a question often asked by parents who face a ten-day course of medication. If there were, life would be a lot simpler. We can give a long-acting shot for a few infections—strep throat, for instance—but this is only because a very low level of antibiotic in the blood is necessary to eradicate the strep germ. In all other infections, a shot three or four times a day would be required to achieve the necessary level of medicine in the blood stream.

Treat all medications seriously, not as candy or as something for which the child is rewarded afterward. Your own firm but gentle manner should indicate that medicine is necessary and you expect the child to cooperate when you administer it.

If medication should be continued after the child is well, a checklist posted on the refrigerator or on an alarm set to ring at the appropriate times may help you to remember. Many liquid medications for children are flavored or sweetened. If your child is old enough to have a few teeth, be sure to follow a bedtime dose with a drink of water and tooth cleaning.

Most children are pretty good about taking medicine, but sometimes you can come across one for whom no amount of cajoling or psychology will work. As an infant, Matthew would kick, scream, and spit at the very sight of a measuring spoon. Whenever medication was really important for Matthew—fortunately, not that often—we would give him a shot initially, and then his mother would do the best she could. I think she donned a wet suit every time she tried to give him medicine. He is now a delightful boy of nine and takes medicine when he must, although reluctantly. Actually, this attitude is probably a healthy one to develop for later life—better, certainly, than thinking that medicine is the answer for all problems. "Tincture of time" is often the best medication for minor problems.

VOMITING AND DIARRHEA

During infancy and childhood, vomiting and diarrhea are common and uncomfortable problems that often occur simultaneously. By vomiting I don't mean spitting up, which is the normal in babies during the first six to nine months. Vomiting is always abnormal. Its onset may be due to motion sickness or because some foods don't agree, but in these cases the vomiting ceases when the motion stops or when the stomach is empty. More serious vomiting, when the baby has an infections or some other intestinal problem, doesn't stop after one episode.

A mild intestinal infection, sometimes accompanied by a fever, is the most common cause of vomiting. Vomiting due to a viral infection will usually last only a day or two. During that time, however, we must watch closely for dehydration. Human beings can live many days without food, but we can only last a short time without fluids. Dehydration in infants and children is more serious than in adults. The younger the child, the less time he or she can survive without replenishing fluids.

Projectile vomiting, a forceful evacuation of stomach contents projecting several feet, is caused by a peculiar coordination between the stomach and the opening at the end of the esophagus. If the baby is not otherwise sick, an occasional episode of projectile vomiting is normal. However, if projectile vomiting persists, especially in a baby one month old, the infant could have pyloric stenosis.

Pyloric stenosis often runs in families, occurs more often in males than females, and is caused by an overgrowth of that portion of the end of the stomach called the pylorus. When the pylorus is too large and too tight, the opening doesn't relax and stomach contents are forced the other way. The treatment of pyloric stenosis is a simple surgical procedure, requiring only a day or two in the hospital. But dehydration is often the more serious problem.

Diarrhea compounds the difficulty with dehydration. Occasional watery stools may be the norm for a breast-fed baby and don't constitute diarrhea. Sometimes breast-fed babies will have as many as ten or twelve small watery stools in twenty-four hours. Problem diarrhea is a combination of frequent, large, and abnormally watery bowel movements. Like vomiting, diarrhea is commonly associated with a viral infection. If vomiting is not present, you can replenish fluid loss in your child more easily. With mild or even moderate diarrhea, a child will not become dehydrated as quickly as with vomiting. While vomiting will cease when the acute infection ends, diarrhea may persist for days or even weeks in a mild form.

The treatment of diarrhea and vomiting involves replacing as much fluid as possible without stimulating further vomiting or diarrhea. Frequently parents make the mistake of trying to feed a child immediately after attacks of vomiting. When I ask how often the child has vomited, they say, "Every time I give him something to eat." Well, stop to think a minute: if the stomach is rejecting food and fluid, the more you put in, the more will come back.

First, allow the stomach to rest for a while. (This could be for six to eight hours for an older child or merely the usual interval between feedings for an infant.) Then start refeeding with clear liquids in small amounts—water, apple juice, clear sodas like 7-UP without the carbonation (let it sit opened, until it goes flat, or warm it slightly). There are also commercial liquids—Pedialyte or Lytren or Infalyte—mixtures of water, salt, and sugar specifically designed to maintain normal fluid and salt balance in babies with upset stomachs. Fruit juices frequently work as laxatives. If a child is experiencing diarrhea along with the vomiting, avoid fruit juices unless you dilute them with water.

Start with just a sip or two of clear liquid, and wait fifteen minutes before you try again. If vomiting subsides, increase the amount to half an ounce. If this stays down for half an hour, try a full ounce. If it all comes back again, wait another half hour and start over.

Similar advice applies to diarrhea. Milk—except for breast milk—and solid foods stimulate the intestines and irritate the bowel, producing more diarrhea. Again, use clear liquids. You don't have to be as careful about the initial amount as when the child is vomiting, although smaller, more frequent feedings are best. When the diarrhea has subsided, don't be in a hurry to reintroduce milk. A child recovering from diarrhea will do best for a few days on bananas, rice or rice cereal, and applesauce. All of these foods have a binding or constipating effect.

Once the acute phase of diarrhea is over, loose stools may persist for as long as four to six weeks. If you continually keep trying to firm up the stools with a diet restricted to constipating foods and clear liquids, you may end up several weeks down the line with a skinny child who still has loose stools. If your child seems to feel well and has one or two loose stools a day, caloric intake is more important.

There are several signs that a child with vomiting and diarrhea is not retaining enough fluid. One is frequency of urination; infants should urinate every two or three hours at least, but with the additional problem of diarrhea, it's sometimes hard to tell if a diapered baby is urinating adequately. A child who is becoming dehydrated won't produce tears when crying, won't have a runny nose, or drool. Your finger if you place it in the child's mouth will feel dry; the tissues around the eyes may become sunken.

If you see any of these signs, call your pediatrician immediately. It's very easy to treat dehydration with intravenous fluid and children recover very quickly.

OTHER COMMON MEDICAL CONDITIONS

Hand-Foot-Mouth Syndrome

The most striking feature of this mild viral infection is the eruption of little blisters on the soles of the feet, on the palms of the hands, and in the mouth. The blisters are white or gray on a red base, are flat, and are generally not painful except in the mouth. The rash generally lasts several days and has no complications, except that a child may be reluctant to eat or take fluids because of the painful mouth lesions. A topical spray such as Chloraspetic used just before eating or drinking may anesthetize the mouth area so that the child can take some fluid. Pieces of chopped-up Popsicle or shaved ice may give pain relief and provide fluid intake.

Pinkeye

Conjunctivitis, or pinkeye, is an inflammation of the tissue covering the eye, caused by either a virus or by bacteria. The condition is usually accompanied by mucus or pus, which causes the eyelids to stick together when the child awakens from sleep. Although some children rub the affected eye, the condition is usually not uncomfortable.

Conjunctivitis responds well to Neosporin, Tobrex, Sodium Sulamyd, or other antibiotic drops, which are, however, not easy to administer to a child who will do everything possible to keep the eyes tightly shut. It's easier if two adults are on hand to do the job: one person to hold the child while the other administers the drops. The usual dose is one drop every four to six hours. If you're not sure a drop went in, repeat the dosage. An extra drop will do no harm—the excess fluid will just overflow.

Conjunctivitis is highly contagious, so wash your hands thoroughly after cleansing an infected eye or administering drops. Use a cotton ball moistened in water to clean the eye, and discard the cotton after use.

If the inflammation hasn't disappeared after three to five days, notify your pediatrician. Sometimes a scratch or foreign body in the eye masquerades as conjunctivitis.

Pinworms

Pinworms are sometimes called threadworms because they look like little pieces of white darning cotton. They live in the lower intestine and come out at night to lay their eggs. They cause itching around the anus, which may awaken a child at night.

Pinworms are contracted from other children, who carry the microscopic eggs around on their fingers and transmit them by direct contact with the child or from the surfaces of shared toys. They are not an indication of a lack of cleanliness of a household but are a very common infection in nursery schools and day-care centers.

Treatment is simple and easy. A child over one year is given a chewable pill (Vermox); one dose is usually all that's necessary. Younger children need a course of liquid medicine for several days. If the pinworms recur, we may treat everyone in the family.

Sheets and pillowcases should be changed when treatment is begun, and the child's fingernails should be kept short and clean.

Eczema

In the past ten years or so there has been a striking increase in the diagnosis of eczema in infants and children. This may be due partly to air pollutants, but it may also be due to the fact that small children have extremely sensitive skin. Drying agents such as soap and water are the major cause of eczema because they remove protective oils and surface layers of skin. Other irritants such as perspiration and indoor air also dry the skin.

Eczema is commonly seen in families with a history of allergy. This doesn't mean that eczema is a specific allergic reation, although certain foods may exacerbate existing excema. It starts most commonly on the inside of the elbows, the backs of the knees and behind the ears, but in small children it may appear anywhere. The affected area may be rough, red, and scaly. Older children will scratch angrily at the itchy rash, but babies who are too young to scratch may just be irritable. Oral antihistamines such as Benadryl may relieve itching.

To alleviate eczema, first minimize the causes of dry skin: bathe the child once every three days or even once a week.

Moisturize the skin with a nonirritating cream or lotion, one without alcohol or fragrance. I recommend Eucerin to my patients.

If the rash is extensive and severe, your pediatrician may prescribe a topical cortisone cream. This is usually very effective but must be used carefully and only as directed. Cortisone cream, used too frequently, can be absorbed into the bloodstream. Cortisone has many side effects, ranging from delayed growth to excessive hair development.

Use a humidifier in the child's room, and dress the child in light clothing to decrease perspiration. Fabrics such as wool and man-made materials such as polyester that do not breathe exacerbate the problem. Cotton knits next to the body are probably best.

Hives

Hives are large, irregular welts that look like huge mosquito bites. Sometimes the cause is obvious: they may come from an allergy to a food or drug. Other causes can be a viral infection or even a strep throat. But most of the time hives just happen. About 80 to 85 percent of the time, we never figure out what brought on the rash, and it never happens again.

Hives start suddenly, and they come and go in various parts of the body. They may be associated with swelling of the eyes and lips, and they often—but not always—itch. If a child has trouble breathing, makes a wheezing sound, or has poor color (pale or bluish), seek medical attention immediately. Such reactions may indicate a life-threatening situation. Most of the time, however, hives merely result in discomfort and look worse than they feel.

If the possible offending substance is something that is easy to avoid, avoid it in the future. If a child is taking an antibiotic when hives appear, we assume that the drug is responsible until proven otherwise.

An antihistamine such as Benadryl or Atarax will control symptoms until the reaction subsides, generally within a week. If the problem is severe or prolonged, your pediatrician may prescribe a short course of oral cortisone.

Impetigo

Impetigo is a bacterial infection of the skin that is common in children of all ages. A small red spot anywhere on the body, but particularly around the face and diaper area, may become a blister which breaks, forming a yellow, honey-colored crust. Scratching or picking at the scab may spread the infection. But even if the child never touches the sore, new lesions may appear around the original one.

Impetigo, as a bacterial infection, almost always requires antibiotics, but there are also local measures that help. Soak the area with a solution of liquid soap such as Hibiclens and warm water until the crust softens, and apply an antibacterial ointment such as Neosporin or Polysporin. The skin will heal more readily if it is exposed to the air. But if your child is in contact with other children, the lesions should be covered to avoid spreading the infection.

Impetigo should begin to heal in three to five days after treatment has begun. If not, your doctor may recommend a change of medication and perhaps take a culture of the lesion to identify the bacteria responsible for the condition.

Ringworm

Ringworm is a fungal infection of the skin that forms a circle with red scaly edges and a clear center. It can start on the arms and legs, the trunk, or the scalp or face, and is probably contracted either from other children or from family pets. It starts slowly and takes weeks to grow larger. This helps to distinguish it from eczema or impetigo, which can look initially similar but progress more rapidly.

For mild cases of ringworm, over-the-counter creams that kill fungus such as Tinactin may be all you need. For more extensive or severe eruptions or conditions that don't respond to over-the-counter medication in a few weeks, prescription cream may be advised. If the infection is widespread or severe, your child may need an oral prescriptive drug. When I have a patient with such a problem, I usually refer the child to a dermatologist for evaluation and treatment.

Scabies

Scabies is a rash caused by a microscopic mite that burrows under the skin. In an older child, the rash appears between the fingers and toes, at the waistline, and on the wrists. In an infant, it may appear on the face, on the bottom of the feet, or on the trunk. The rash can take many forms—blisters, red bumps, or raised streaks—and may mimic impetigo and eczema.

The scabies organism is readily transmitted by humans and animals, and can live for long periods of time on household surfaces such as bed linens and toys. To avoid spread we advise parents to wash the child's bedding, clothing, and toys. Not everyone who has been in contact with scabies develops a rash, but other members of the family may become infected.

There are several preparations used to treat scabies, most commonly Eurax and Kwell, both prescription drugs. The cream or lotion is applied to the skin for several hours and then washed off. The medications are safe when used as directed; but using them too often, especially on broken skin, can lead to toxic side effects. So use them only as your doctor prescribes. The rash may take a week or more to fade, but there should be no new lesions after you use the medicine. Occasionally a second application becomes necessary.

For reasons that remain obscure, scabies has reached epidemic proportions in the pediatric population. Fortunately most children have lifelong immunity after one eruption.

NINE

Safety

THROUGHOUT THIS BOOK, I've been urging parents to relax and trust their own instincts. But parents must not relax when it comes to a child's safety. Children have the boundless capacity to turn everyday objects into previously unrecognized hazards. Caring for an infant or a toddler means constant vigilance and frequent checking and rechecking of your environment, both at home and outside.

Some minor accidents are, of course, inevitable: bangs, bumps, and cuts are a part of natural development. But many major accidents could be prevented if parents had only thought ahead. In all fairness, however, babies and children can create situations you never dreamed could happen. Most could have been avoided if parents exercised foresight and common sense, and were aware of what a child can do at different stages of development.

From birth to four months, watch out for things within a baby's reach, and prevent falls from surfaces such as changing tables or the top of your bed. Just because a baby hasn't learned to roll over doesn't mean that it's safe to leave the baby in the middle of your king-sized bed and turn away. Babies wriggle and squirm, and can cover amazing distances in a short time. I tell parents of small infants to place the child on the floor if they must turn away for a moment. It's impossible to fall off the floor.

Between four and nine months, drawers, cabinets, and surfaces less than eighteen inches off the floor are fair game for a crawling infant. Clear off coffee tables, and move precious possessions to upper drawers.

From nine to eighteen months, toddlers attack anything within sight and reach—from houseplants to electrical cords. Unplug your curling iron and put it away when it's not in use, and remove any liquid cosmetics (anything that can be drunk) from the bathroom counters.

After eighteen months, toddlers start to use drawers and chairs for ladders and can break and enter into anything, including medicine cabinets. Don't count on bottles being "childproof." Toddlers also start imitating adult behavior and may try to start the washer or dryer, or turn on the stove.

Basic principles for protecting your child are these: first, take care of all potential hazards the instant you are aware of them—not tomorrow or just after you answer the phone or doorbell. Second, don't assume that what was safe *yesterday* is still safe today; check and recheck everything in your dwelling, from the previously clean floor to the previously unfrayed electrical cords. Third, nothing is completely out of a child's reach. A determined toddler can manage any childproof lock or scale any domestic Everest to reach something attractive. Finally, realize that all the safety devices you can buy, from childproof locks to child-resistant medicine bottles, are not just a substitute for adult vigilance; a safety device only slows down a child so an adult has a better chance to get there in time.

When I made this statement to the parents of an eighteen-month-old boy, they nodded knowingly. They had recently discovered him in another room, having not only removed all the plug covers from all the sockets, but in the process of choking and gagging on one that he had put into his mouth.

Accidents are more likely to occur at certain times—when parents are tired or diverted by the phone or absorbed in their own discussions. Accidents also occur when assumptions are made: the other parent is watching the child; what was safe yesterday is safe today. A mother of four girls arrived at my office with her youngest child, who had fallen out of her corduroy baby carrier when the strap broke. After examining the child and reassuring the mother that everything was all right, we discussed the accident. The mother was angry that the strap could have broken and was going to write to the manufacturer. But when I asked how long she had had it, she paused for a moment and sheepishly said, "It's been used for three other babies." Obviously, even the safest, best-built equipment doesn't last forever.

With these basic principles in mind, I'd like to lead you through a systematic plan for preparedness, with specific suggestions for all the areas of your life and home.

ANTICIPATING EMERGENCIES

Post a list of emergency information near every phone in the house. (If an emergency occurs upstairs, the list near the kitchen phone is of little use.) On each list, write or print your own name and address and the name of your child in large letters. Many people don't think clearly during emergencies. In your absence, a babysitter or visitors to your house may need this help.

In addition, write down the name and phone number of a neighbor who has agreed to be a contact. List the phone numbers of the police, the fire department, the paramedics, the local hospital's emergency room, the poison center, and your pediatrician and adult doctor.

Familiarize yourself with emergency measures. My best advice is to take a first-aid and cardiopulmonary-resuscitation (CPR) course at the local YMCA, Red Cross, or community hospital. If you know what to do in an emergency, you will avoid panic and you may save a life.

Install smoke detectors in the hallway near bedrooms and inside the entrance to each bedroom. Keep a fire extinguisher in the kitchen and on the second floor if there are two stories in your house. The ABC type of extinguisher is good for all types of household fires. Remember that the usual type of household extinguisher will spray about ten or fifteen seconds. If a fire occurs, spray the base of the fire, not the top of the flames.

Always call the fire department, even if you think the fire is out and the danger is past.

Rehearse a fire-escape plan for the family periodically. If you live in a two-story house and there is no easy exit to the roof, invest in some fold-up ladders. These are available at hardware stores. Buy as many as necessary, and keep them under the windows that you've decided are the best escape routes. If you have more than one child, decide which parent will be responsible for which child, and designate a family meeting place outside the house.

Contact your local fire station for written information about fire safety and possible escape routes in your house. Revise the plan as you make changes in your home. A large piece of furniture may obstruct a previous escape route, or bedroom assignments may change from one year to another.

Make sure that all children's nightwear you buy or receive is flame retardant.

Instruct babysitters about your safety precautions. Provide babysitters with instructions to be followed in an emergency. Walk through the house, pointing out the fire extinguishers, operation of locks, and how the latches work on the windows. This is especially important if the sitter is a teenager. Sitters should have no visitors, and phone calls should be discouraged. The babysitter's attention should be on your child.

Increase safety by buying items with childproof caps. Childproof caps have not eliminated the problem of medicine and product ingestion, but they have been responsible for lowering the incidence of serious poisonings. Whenever possible, always buy an item with the childproof top.

Pay special attention to small objects that can be swallowed. Children put everything in their mouths. Swallowing a parent's contact lens may not constitute a major accident, but a small disk battery, if ingested, can cause serious gastrointestinal problems or obstruct a child's airway.

Keep ipecac on hand. When your child starts to crawl, ask your pediatrician whether you should have a bottle of ipecac at home. Some pharmacies will provide ipecac at no cost if prescribed by a doctor. Ipecac induces vomiting, useful if a child has eaten or drunk something that can safely be removed from the stomach by the vomiting process.

Before using ipecac, check with your pediatrician or the poison center as to whether or not it's safe and appropriate to give the ipecac for the particular material your child has ingested. Some substances, such as drain cleaners, can do further damage on the way back up and have to be dealt with in special ways.

ROOM-BY-ROOM SAFETY MEASURES

In *Baby Proofing Your Home,* Mike Hayward defines "Baby Primitive Decor" as "a tasteful learning experience in clean interior lines and uncluttered open spaces." Hayward goes on to advise parents to remove all portable articles from table tops and counters. This includes knick-knacks, cigarette lighters, vases, small glass dishes, and so forth. An essential part of this décor includes corner guards to pad the sharp edges of furniture. You won't find yourself saying "No!" so often if your house contains a minimum number of objects that might cause trouble.

To babyproof your house, crawl on your hands and knees as though you were crawling through the jungle on a guerrilla mission. Forget about looking at things from your adult point of view. Consider everything as a child would, as objects to be played with. Consider the temptation of drapery cords, and think of all that could be done with them. Examine electrical outlets behind tables. Look with your child's eyes at the plants, and see them as possible food. All houseplants can be considered toxic, although some are more toxic than others: Dieffenbachia, for example, can paralyze the throat. Once you have a crawling infant, all houseplants should be out of reach or out of the house.

Relocate heavy pieces of furniture so that they obstruct electrical outlets. If you can't barricade all of the outlets, buy safety covers or safety plugs for those that are exposed. The best kind are spring-loaded devices that require a difficult turning and pushing motion to be plugged in.

Remember that all these gadgets only delay the time it takes a child to get into trouble. None is a substitute for parental watchfulness. If wires travel along the floor, tack them to a baseboard to keep them away from little hands and mouths.

Baby primitive décor excludes tablecloths. These can be pulled down with regularity as a child tries to stand and the possible emergencies are obvious.

Mommy's or other women's purses can be treasure troves of dangerous articles, since most of them contain nail files, other small sharp objects, or even medications. Don't leave purses on the floor.

Having crawled around the floor once, your job is not done. Circumstances are continually changing. Check periodically for objects that may be embedded in the carpet and for appliances whose plugs and cords are within reach.

Kitchen

Think of the kitchen as a serious work area, and remember that a stove, for all its benefits, is a dangerous appliance. I recently treated an eighteen month old and her mother for minor burns on the hands and arms when a double boiler unexpectedly blew up. Avoid such an emergency by placing your child in a playpen in the dining area visible from the kitchen or in the farthest corner of the kitchen.

Make the same journey in the kitchen on your hands and knees to see what's accessible to a crawling child. One-third of all accidental poisonings occur in the kitchen. More than half are the result of cleaning products, such as bleach, detergents, drain cleaners, furniture polish, insecticides, and oven cleaners, as well as flavored children's vitamins, which are often kept in the kitchen. Children don't taste before they swallow, so don't assume that smell or taste will be a deterrent.

Use childproof locks even if you think your child can't reach the cabinet in which you've stored dangerous material. A determined child will find a way to get to it.

If your kitchen trash can is out in the open, be careful of what you put there. An energetic child can remove anything that you discard. If you keep the trash can locked and under the sink, you will keep your baby from exploring the trash as well as throwing away your keys—a not uncommon occurrence.

Be sure that cups containing hot liquid are in the center of the table, and forget about tablecloths that can be pulled off of table tops. Keep appliance cords far back on kitchen counters.

If you use oven or drain cleaner, don't buy the economy size. These agents are so deadly that with a child in the house it's false economy. Buy a single-use size, and discard the container after you use it, even if the can is not empty.

Don't ever put cleaning substances or other chemicals into food containers. A child can mistake such a substance for food; and adults have been known to feed a child a chemical, assuming that the contents of the container were edible. Before feeding anything to a child from a container that you haven't just opened yourself, smell and taste the contents first.

Be careful about irons. A child can be burned by even

momentary contact with a hot iron. Never let a child play in a room where someone is ironing. Make sure that the iron is cool if you need to leave the room to put the laundry away.

With all the dangerous areas of the kitchen, your child needs permission to occupy at least a small part of it to be near family activity. Designate a cabinet or low drawer as your child's special place, and fill it with Tupperware or old pots and pans that can be used as toys. This provides a diversion from forbidden territory and a recognized place for the child.

Bathrooms

Bathroom locks are a major potential hazard. For most bathroom doors, you need only a small screwdriver or coat hanger to release the lock from the outside. Practice this procedure before your child is accidentally locked in the bathroom, so you know how to release the lock when you have to.

Appliances in the bathrooms, especially curling irons that can burn small fingers, are the cause of many visits to my office. After use, put all electrical appliances in a safe cupboard out of a child's reach. Of course, all bottles and jars in the bathroom should be plastic. And be sure to leave the lid of the toilet seat down.

As for toilet paper, most children love to pull it off the roll. Put a rubber band around the roll; it will still be accessible to you, and you won't spend your time rerolling miles of toilet paper.

Take a close look at your medicine cabinet, and throw out any prescription medication not in current use or out of date. The chance of needing the same prescription again before it expires is so slim and the chance of the baby climbing up and taking it is so great, that it makes no sense to keep it around. As emphasized earlier, all medications should have childproof tops. Whatever pills you're not using should be flushed down the toilet rather than thrown in the trash.

Discard any over-the-counter medications you don't use regularly. Ben Gay and other deep-heat preparations, for example, are highly toxic when ingested. If you suddenly have a sore back, it's better to take a hot shower or to use a heating pad than to keep such a potentially dangerous medication around.

One of my colleagues at UCLA came home to discover something that makes a pediatrician's blood run cold. His policy has been to keep all medications in a tackle box with a padlock, and he hid the key on a bathroom shelf. However, his two-year-old son saw where the key was hidden, opened the box, and was passing out medications to the children in the neighborhood, playing doctor like his daddy. The moral to the story is obvious: the only truly safe storage for drugs and other items—perfume and nail-polish remover, for example—is in a fishing tackle box with a combination lock. Note the combination on the box with nail polish or paint. Your child can't possibly figure out the numbers. But, as you can see, even a padlock with a key is not childproof.

If you're administering medication to a child, read and reread the instructions on the label, and do this under a good light. A parent-induced poisoning is a terrible tragedy. Never keep medication in a child's bedroom. It should be securely stored in the bathroom.

All medicines should be treated with respect. If children get the idea that medicine is candy or that one is rewarded for taking it, they are more likely to experiment on their own. Deal with medicine matter-of-factly, as something that must be taken when it's needed but without reward or other hullabaloo.

Bedrooms

Survey what you keep on top of your dresser. Perfumes are drinkable and medications edible. Be sure that bottom drawers have contents that present no risks—socks or sweaters rather than small items such as buttons or coins.

Windows in All Rooms

All windows should be securely screened and should have window guards that will not open more than a few inches. The kind that open from the top are safer than those that open from the bottom. Furniture should be moved away from the windows, especially on upper floors, since a child may be tempted to climb up and out.

Stairs

If there are stairs in your house, put gates across both the top and bottom, and don't forget the basement stairs. It's clear that children on the upper floor can tumble down, but people forget that infants on a lower floor can crawl up and then fall down.

Check the width of railings on stairways, especially wrought iron railings. I've treated a number of children who slipped through railings and fell to the floor below. If you find that the railings are too wide, block them with a sheet of plastic or plywood until your child is too large to slip or squeeze through.

CHILD-CARE EQUIPMENT AND SAFETY

Cribs

The side slats of a crib should be no farther apart than 2⅜ inches. Round slats are better than square ones, which are more easily chewed into splinters. Make sure the mattress on the crib fits tightly. Gaps between mattress and frame can trap an infant or small baby. Push the mattress firmly in all directions; the space created between mattress and crib should be no less than 1 inch. The devices locking the sides of the crib should be strong, should be babyproof, and should have no sharp edges.

Some cribs come equipped with bumper pads. The best are the kind that attach with snappers. If they tie, be sure the strings are short and tied on the outside of the crib so that they're out of baby's reach. Inspect the bumper pads regularly for rips and tears that invite exploration by little fingers.

Once a child can stand, remove all large stuffed animals and bumper pads from the crib. These can provide a handy foothold and can perhaps cause an unfortunate tumble.

If you buy a secondhand crib, make sure that the paint is not lead-based. If there's no way to determine this, sand the crib and repaint it.

Dangling gyms that hang over the crib should be removed as soon as the baby starts to sit up. If the crib is near a window, watch for hanging drapery cords. Either tie the cords up so that they're out of baby's reach, or move the crib away from them. Fancy cribs and cradles with cutouts and curlicues make nice heirlooms, but babies can trap their heads in them. I recommend buying the simplest and plainest crib, even if it's not the most beautiful.

Infant Seats

These are convenient for transporting the baby who is not walking, but be sure that the seat is sturdy and well padded, and that the seat belt is always fastened. Many babies can arch their backs and throw themselves out of the seat if the belt is not securely attached. Check the supporting rods in the back of the chair regularly; wear and tear weakens them, and the seat may collapse.

Don't think of an infant seat as a substitute babysitter. I've treated many babies who toppled off a counter top or table top onto the floor, even when secured in their infant seats. If you must leave the room, place the baby in the seat on the floor. And never use the infant seat as a car seat. It won't provide the proper restraint if an accident occurs.

High Chairs

Sturdily built, noncollapsible high chairs are always safer than collapsible ones, which can trap small fingers and may indeed collapse if their connections are not fully secured. Select a chair with nonskid rubber caps on the legs, and test it carefully in the store before purchasing it. Push the chair around, and jiggle it as a vigorous toddler would. Any chair you buy should have a seat belt. Always use the crotch strap as well as the seat belt to prevent the child from sliding under the tray and onto the floor. Don't permit your child to stand up in the chair, and never leave a toddler unattended. If you must answer the phone, take the child and chair to a location near the phone.

Walkers

Walkers are popular because they allow a nonwalking infant increased mobility as well as a play surface that's in constant reach. However, walkers are also a major cause of serious head injuries. The wheels on a walker may catch on the edge of a carpet and catapult the child, who's usually moving at breakneck speed. In addition, the danger of a walker anywhere near a stairway is obvious. If my patients ask my advice before buying a walker, I usually recommend against it.

OUTDOOR SAFEGUARDS

Your backyard, though it may be the most pleasant place in the world, is fraught with danger for an infant or a small child. Things that are growing there are your first concern. Immediately pull out the mushrooms that pop up after a rain. Oleander bushes, a favorite planting in my area, are poisonous and should be removed if a family has young children. Snail pellets in the roses find their way into children's mouths.

Keep children away from the lawn mower at all times. This is an absolute no-no, whether the mower is running or not. These are powerful machines and have often caused serious injuries, from amputations to eye injuries, in children.

Treat all bodies of water, from wading pools to fish ponds, as you would a swimming pool. Remove water from wading pools when they're not being used, and don't let a small child near any water unless an older person is present. Even two inches of water presents a hazard.

Someone must always be in charge of a child in the area of a swimming pool. If the person in charge has to leave even for a moment, another adult must take over and must acknowledge that that responsibility is accepted. This may sound like a military operation, but drownings and near-drownings have occurred when adults were under the impression that someone else was watching a child. Never let another child be responsible for a baby.

The final hazard of the outdoors is the sun. Children are especially susceptible to sunburn since their skin is translucent and doesn't have all the protective layers of dead cells and thickened skin that we develop later. A baby even with an umbrella and a hat can still suffer a significant burn from the reflected glare on water and concrete. The only sure preventive for sunburn is an effective sunscreen. If your baby is light-complexioned, a sunscreen whose label reads 15 or 19 is necessary. For children with darker skins, a lesser strength may be adequate. But even light-skinned black children may burn after too much exposure to sun.

Sunscreens work best if applied half an hour before exposure. They should be reapplied at frequent intervals, especially if the baby goes into water.

TOY SAFETY

An entire book could be written about toy safety. There are more than 150,000 toys that need to be surveyed for safety, and not all of them are—or can be—carefully monitored. So it's up to a parent to make the final judgment.

Make sure that the eyes on stuffed animals are embroidered and not sewn on like buttons, for the latter can easily come off and be swallowed. Check any stuffed toys periodically for rips and tears, and repair or replace the toys as necessary. If the child is particularly attached to a certain stuffed animal, there are always surgical procedures you can devise to keep the object safe without destroying its identity.

Inspect all toys before purchasing them. Pull all the parts, and twist firmly. Infants and toddlers can easily choke on toy parts. In addition, toys should be sufficiently large so that they can't fit into a child's mouth. You may have noticed that teething rings and rattles of recent manufacture no longer have handles because handles can become lodged in the back of a child's mouth. A few years ago, I x-rayed a child with severe wheezing. The x-ray revealed a foreign body in the lung, which turned out to be the foot of a foam-rubber doll. The child had twisted it off, but the mother hadn't even realized it was missing.

The toys of older children that might be dangerous for the younger ones should be kept separate. Lego parts, for example, can easily be eaten by or can cause choking in an infant. An older child should be aware of safety precautions for a younger sibling and should be monitored frequently for compliance.

Toy chests must not have heavy lids that are dangerous if they snap shut on fragile necks. If someone wants to make a toy chest for your child, request that it have no lid.

Even balloons can be dangerous for infants and toddlers. Don't allow your child to play with balloons that are not inflated. If an inflated balloon bursts, be sure to gather up all the scraps of rubber. Infants, with their sharp teeth, should not be allowed to chew on balloons.

FIRST AID FOR MINOR ACCIDENTS

A number of injuries and accidents are unavoidable in childhood. Here's what to do in the first minutes if the following accidents occur.

Burns

The burned area must be cooled immediately. If hot liquid has caused the burn, remove the child's clothing as fast as you can. Plunge the burned area into cold water, or apply a cold, wet washcloth. Keep the area cool for at least fifteen minutes after the burn has occurred.

Once you've started cooling measures, call your pediatrician. Some areas of the body need special treatment in order to prevent later problems. A burn on the edge of the mouth, for example, may heal with a cosmetic deformity, or a burn on the palm of the hand can heal in such a way that a finger is permanently bent. A child's skin is extremely delicate and thin. A minor burn for an adult can be more serious in an infant and may need more extensive treatment.

Don't apply creams, first-aid sprays, butter, or any greasy substance to burned areas. Wait for your doctor's advice. Go to the emergency room of your nearest hospital if you can't reach your doctor.

Although some of the burns I've treated have looked pretty severe at first, children heal so beautifully that most minor burns leave no scars at all.

Cuts

The treatment for all cuts is the same: apply pressure directly over the wound to stop the bleeding. Lacerations in certain areas, such as the head or tongue, can cause profuse bleeding out of proportion to the severity of the injury. When the bleeding stops, the cut may turn out to be a tiny wound buried in the hair or a little nick on the edge of the tongue.

If you think the laceration may need stitches, there's no need to endanger life and limb by rushing to the doctor or emergency room. There's plenty of time to stitch up a wound; as long as it's taken care of within a few hours, it will heal just fine.

Head Injuries

A child's head takes the brunt of most falls. Because of the rich blood supply to the scalp, a bang on the head may raise a good-sized bump in a few seconds. Most infants and toddlers won't allow you to hold a cold cloth on the bump to decrease the size of the swelling, so it's futile to try. If the bump is several inches across, however, or continues to swell even after the injury, there may be a skull fracture underneath. Call your pediatrician in that case.

If the child cries for a few minutes and then goes about business as usual, there's probably no need for concern, even if a good-sized bump appears. But if the child seems lethargic within the next few hours, stumbles more than usual, vomits, or exhibits any unusual behavior, call your pediatrician.

There is a widespread misunderstanding that someone with a head injury shouldn't be allowed to fall asleep. That makes no sense, especially if it's bedtime or naptime. Just check the child every hour to make sure there isn't any vomiting and that the child can be roused. Of course, if a child loses consciousness, even only briefly, the doctor should be called immediately.

Nosebleeds

In children, most nosebleeds originate from the front of the nose on the wall, or septum, dividing the nostrils. Forget all the old wives' tales about applying ice to the back of the neck, placing garlic under the chin, or putting brown paper under the nose, all of which my patients have tried. To stop the bleeding, apply pressure directly to the bleeding site by pinching the nostrils. Bring the child to a sitting position, and firmly grasp the nostrils between your thumb and first finger, letting go after five minutes to check if the bleeding has stopped. Tell a story or sing a song to make the time pass for the child.

Sometimes nosebleeds occur after trauma, sometimes they are the result of a dry, irritated nose from having taken decongestants, and sometimes they happen for no discernible reason.

If a child has repeated nosebleeds, children's nose drops such as Pediatric Afrin or Neo-Synephrine for infants may be administered for a few nights. These cause the small blood vessels to constrict and the lining of the nose to heal more quickly. A humidifier at night may help prevent the nasal membranes from drying out and bleeding again. Sometimes I advise my patients to apply a little Vaseline just inside the nose for a few nights to lubricate the membranes so they can heal.

CAR SAFETY

Car accidents have caused more casualties in this country than all the wars in our history. The overwhelming majority of these deaths and injuries would not have occurred if adults and children had been properly restrained.

Tennessee was the first state to pass a law requiring all children to be restrained in safe car seats. Originally, children could be held on an adult's lap, but the law was strengthened when legislators realized that an adult's lap affords no protection when an accident occurs. Subsequently, car-seat use in Tennessee rose from 8 percent to over 30 percent, and the death rate for children in car accidents decreased by more than 50 percent. Car seats and seat belts really do save lives, and now all states have passed similar laws.

Laws are effective only if they are observed and enforced. The arguments for not using seat belts and car seats are based on misinformation and are usually complete nonsense.

Some people think that it's safe to hold a child on their lap while riding in a car. When a car that has been traveling 30 miles per hour crashes, a child can be thrown with the force of 500 pounds. Even Arnold Schwarzenegger can't hold onto a 500-pound projectile.

Another specious objection is "I use seat belts on the highway, but not for short trips." The majority of accidents occur on local roads close to home, and the major single factor responsible for car accidents—the drunk driver—is on every road at all times. Also, although highways have cars going at higher speeds, local roads have opposing traffic, stop lights, and left turns, all of which increase the possibility of accidents.

People who want to resist seat-belt use claim that their Uncle Harry would have died had he not been thrown free of a crash. There's usually little truth to this. Most injuries occur because people are thrown about inside or outside the car. Children and adults are much more likely to survive if they use car seats and seat belts.

There are four types of seats: infant carriers, which are useful only for children up to 20 pounds; toddler seats for children from 20 to 40 pounds; convertible seats, which can be used for both infants and toddlers; and booster seats, only for children over 40 pounds. Although the convertible seat may cost almost twice as much as an infant carrier, in the long run it may be more economical because you only need to buy one seat. However, the infant carrier is easier and lighter for carrying out of the car.

There are 47 car seats that meet federal highway safety standards. Twenty-seven of these are approved by the FAA for use in aircraft as well. The following car seats are approved for both cars and airplanes:

The Century Infant Love Seat and the Century 100, 200, and 300 Car Seats

Cosco-Peterson First Ride (models 582 and 682), Safe-T-Seat, Luxury Safe-T-Seat, Safe-T-Shield, Safe and Easy, Safe-n-Snug (models 323 and 423), Safe-T-Mate (models 378 and 478), Travel Hi-Lo, Deluxe Travel Hi-Lo (models 183 and 283), and the Deluxe High Back Travel Hi-Lo (models 383 and 483)

Pride Tumble Pride Ride (models 820 and 830)

Strolee Wee Care (models 599, 612, and 618) and Wee Care Auto Booster (models 602 and 604)

If you buy a secondhand seat, the instructions and factory information may be missing. If so, write to the manufacturer to be sure that you're using the seat correctly—some seats need a tether strap anchored in the back window, for example; and if you buy a second hand seat without the strap, it is hardly safe.

Infants should ride facing backward because that's the safest position. Older children face front once their legs are too long to sit backward. Also, older children need to see out of the window if they are to be content when restrained on a long car ride. The back seat is safest, although an infant may ride facing backward in the front seat.

The specific car seat you use must be compatible with the car or cars you will be driving. Be sure to test the seat in your own car before you buy it. For example, some seat belt buckles are too thick to pass through some frames, or some belts are too short, and some cars have low bucket seats that are too short for the bases of some car seats.

Some bright toddlers of, say, eighteen months, figure out how partially to unhook car seats and wiggle out of them. You should react to this as though the child had run into the street. Pull off the road, and stop the car. Make a federal case out of it while you resecure the child. Some mischief is a misdemeanor and some is felonious, and this qualifies as a felony. Car safety should be important to you, and your child will soon learn to respect the restrictions.

My final word on this topic is to remember that children imitate their parents. If you always wear a seat belt whenever you're in a car, your child will follow your lead. You can't be a relaxed and competent parent if you're not alive and well. You and anyone you care about must never travel without proper restraints.

TEN

Gourmet Babies and Your Baby

THE MATURATION DERBY

THERE'S NO WAY a parent can escape the barrage of material about the amazing learning potential of infants. Literature from such organizations as the Better Baby Institute in Philadelphia shows you how to teach math to your one year old, how to teach your baby not only to play a musical instrument but to compose music. The modern prophets of "superdevelopment" even say that "your baby can become an expert in gymnastics, ballet, swimming, or whatever physical skills you desire." The worst part is they claim that you can make any baby into a "superb human being."

Why does this drive me crazy? Because it gives the message to parents and, more importantly to children, that they have to *do* something in order to be acceptable. In other words, children are not wonderful, superb human beings simply because they are alive. In an article in the *Chicago Sun Times,* Tom McNamee quotes a mother in an affluent Chicago suburb as saying to her child, "I don't want to love you just because you are. You have to *do* something."

It's not surprising that parents want to give children the necessary tools to succeed in a world where it seems as though winning is everything. This in itself isn't bad, but it can be carried to extremes. Many parents feel guilty when they don't live up to the prescriptions of the experts. One of my patients attended the Better Baby Institute course and said: "On the way home from each class, I started feeling that my son had missed the boat. But when I got back to the real world, I found I didn't have a problem."

Common sense and perspective are necessary. Claims of the new learning programs are likely to be sensational, and you should take them with a grain of salt. The truth is, starting from the first day of life, babies learn an incredible amount without extra stimulation. Like animals and birds, babies and young children learn naturally. There is very little that can deter children from learning or keep them from learning in their own way and at their own pace.

The push to accelerate development can be harmful. It would seem that teaching infants to swim is not only an enjoyable experience but a good thing in terms of safety. However, large quantities of water can be swallowed, causing a dilution of sodium in the blood stream and subsequent seizures. In addition, the pool water must be kept very warm; and the warmer the water, the more germs survive despite chlorination. Several types of infections have spread easily among infants in swim classes.

There are drawbacks to gym classes for babies as well. If children under a year are taught to hang by their arms, problems in their joints can result. In other words, there's likely to be a negative as well as a positive side to all these activities.

Some of the highly publicized theories are simply based on false information. About fifteen years ago, it was claimed that reading problems and learning disabilities could be traced to a faulty developmental sequence. Children who had difficulty reading, it was said, went directly from sitting to walking, omitting the stage of crawling. Their learning difficulties could be overcome by returning to precrawling days and correcting the sequence. There was no scientific basis for this theory, but people still ask me if a child who fails to crawl will have problems.

Crawling is not a necessary developmental milestone. Some of the smartest children I know displayed the most bizarre methods of locomotion before walking. Some roll over and over, and one little girl sat in a half-lotus position and scooted backward wherever she wanted to go.

Certainly, informed and attentive parents have a significant influence on a child's development. Dr. Judy Howard at UCLA found that babies in a responsive family environment showed superior development compared to those in homes where parents spent less time with them. We also know that the first child in a family, who usually receives more attention than the second, often talks sooner. He or she is not necessarily smarter, but learns faster.

The I.Q. of normal children within the same family is in the same general range no matter what special attention one child or the other may receive. The effect of additional environmental stimulation on normal children is very subtle. A parent can stimulate love of learning and a curiosity about the world, but only if the parent already has that curiosity. Imagine the future of a child my husband observed in the hospital cafeteria one Sunday while he was waiting for me. The child, a three-year-old girl, had interrupted her parents to ask, "What color is this chair?" Her mother tapped her on the arm and said, "Drink your juice." If this exchange was typical, the child was not receiving the message that the world is interesting, that curiosity and the joy of learning enrich our lives.

I had a different kind of experience coming back from San Francisco, when I was seated next to a woman and her small son. We had to wait at the airline terminal while take-off was delayed, and I watched the little boy get hungry and bored. After exhausting the supply of diversions and toys in her carry-on bag, the mother took out the card describing the emergency exits and started to ask the child how many blue things he could find, then how many round things he saw. The child was quietly distracted, and the time went quickly. He was learning something new in an interesting way. I daresay he will have an easier and more interesting time later in life than the other child.

My husband calls the current obsession with child development the "maturation derby." He's talking about parents who are always making comparisons between their child and other children. These adults don't feel they are "good" unless their child can perform as well as or better than the other children. Some parents are already anxious about the competition in nursery school. It's natural to compare your child with others of the same age, but remember that the child who walks or talks earlier is not necessarily more intelligent than the one who does so later. One of my patients was in a social group when all the mothers started urging their babies to display their accomplishments. One mother urged her baby to say "Bye bye"; another demonstrated the cute faces her baby would make on command. My patient became so frustrated that when her turn came she said to her child, "Sit up and beg."

Another example of overdoing the maturation derby occurred when I saw a one-year-old patient for the first time. When I asked the mother if the child said "Mamma" or "Dada" yet, she replied proudly, that not only did her child say those words, but also "older sister," and "pencil," and a number of other words that one year olds rarely have at their command. I asked further questions and discovered that the mother and father were professors of linguistics and knew many languages, including Mandarin, Cantonese, Kurdish, and Sanskrit. When the child uttered a combination of sounds, they could often find a word in one or another language that contained those sounds. I named a syndrome after them: Acute Parental Overinterpretation.

All this is not to say that you shouldn't be informed about childhood development and take advantage of some of the educational opportunities available to you. At the same time, a child needs to explore the world on an individual basis. The problem with all the enrichment programs is the implication that every waking moment should be directed toward some specific learning goal. The truth is, children are wonderfully creative about learning things on their own. Children need to learn to be self-sufficient and to entertain themselves. Ultimately, these children are easier for parents to care for.

When my patient Tatiana was between one and two, she seemed irritable, tired, and cranky much of the time. I was somewhat surprised at this behavior, because she had been a pleasant, easy baby. Some months later, she seemed her old self again. I asked what had changed, and Tatiana's mother, who is a teacher, said, "I used to come home from work and take Tati to museums, park programs, all around the city—to make up for the fact that I hadn't been with her all day. Then I realized that life doesn't have to be a field trip. Once I let her play quietly—as long as she knew I was there—she was much happier and more relaxed."

Another one of my mothers brought her two and a half year old to me because she was tired all the time. The child would wake up in the morning and say, "Mommy, I'm broken."

Further questioning revealed that this child was enrolled in at least one program every day, sometimes two, from nursery school to ballet to art classes to whatever else her well-intentioned mother could find. When I suggested that perhaps the child was being asked to do too much, her mother said, "But I don't want her to miss anything." I pointed out that the child was missing the most important part of childhood, and that letting her have some "free time" was more important than all the classes she could attend. At her next visit, the mother had eliminated about half the child's activities, and both of them were feeling better.

Parents need to ask themselves: What are our goals in child rearing? Do we want a child to be a successful corporate officer who works ninety hours a week, never sees the family, and is featured in *Fortune*? If I may speak for all of us, I think we really want to raise children who are able to realize their goals and maintain their self-esteem no matter what they choose to do.

The roots of success are certainly planted in early life, but that doesn't include pushing and shoving for early achievement. Rebecca's mother called to ask me if I would write a letter of recommendation for application to an exclusive private school some distance away. I know that children grow up faster than we think, but it seemed to me that Rebecca was still too young to attend school. When I pulled her chart from the file, I saw that my memory was not failing: she was only two and a half.

In an article in the *New York Times,* Susan Strautberg has critical words to say about a nursery-school prep course designed to prepare toddlers for entry to the "best" nursery schools. Of 800 applicants to one school, I can only think of the built-in disappointment of the 770 rejects for the 30 places in the class. A child who has barely begun to walk is already failing in parents' eyes.

Yes, this is a competitive world. But remember that there are two other *C*'s besides competition: cooperating and caring. Learning to play *with* other children is more important than learning to play *better than* other children. Being secure in your parents' love and approval is more important than proving you are a superior child.

Let your child be a child.

FANCY TOYS AND EQUIPMENT

A new mother asked me once for a list of all the toys she should buy for her child at each stage of development. When I asked why, she said, "I don't want to leave out any toy my daughter should have. She may miss something."

Having been raised in a somewhat Spartan household, I remember the longing I felt for expensive toys, and as an adult, I've enjoyed buying presents for the children in my life. Too much is not good, however. One Christmas several years ago, my husband and I stopped at Diana's house. Diana was the first child born in a circle of friends, and everyone arrived with arms full of Christmas presents. My husband and I, with a shopping bag overflowing with gifts, were no exception. Diana was seated on the living room floor, surrounded by toys of all sizes and description. "How are you, Diana?" I asked.

The little girl sighed and said, "I have *too many* toys." She was overwhelmed by the sheer quantity, and unable—at least temporarily—to enjoy any of them.

Everyday household objects can often be as stimulating and effective as elaborate, expensive toys. Infants love to play with empty Tupperware containers. They'll throw them, chew them, put things in, take things out, and use them for anything their imaginations conjure up. For toddlers, a large box or carton serves as a train, car, hideaway, or playhouse. Some children even prefer the containers in which toys are shipped to the contents themselves. The best toys are those toys that have the least structure, that do the least themselves. A child's imagination then has free rein.

Also, there's no way to know what object or toy a child will treasure. My favorite childhood toy was a ball of yarn. It was an ugly color—variegated maroon and brown—but I thought that ball of yarn was beautiful and created all sorts of fantasy objects with it. I did have a large lifelike doll, but didn't play with her very often and preferred my yarn ball. I often see infants feeling, tasting, turning, and banging the plastic nipple covers from their bottles while more decorative rattles and stuffed dogs are ignored.

Carol, now an adult and my editor, was given many dolls with elaborate wardrobes as a child. But they never much appealed to her. She put them all in a doll crib, covered them with a blanket and said they had measles. Her favorite toy was an empty tooth-powder can. When she lost it on an automobile trip, her father had to scour a city for another before she could go to sleep.

I feel the same way about fancy children's equipment as I do about toys. Some of the new equipment may be of the "can't live without" kind. Sassy Seats, for example, are brilliantly designed and allow parents to tote their children anywhere, including restaurants. A Sassy Seat attaches to the side of a table and is held in place by the weight of the child. This is one piece of equipment that I recommend, but be sure the top of the table is firmly anchored to the base and that the table is heavy enough to support the child, or baby and seat may topple over, bringing the table down with them.

At the same time, a $50 lambskin, claiming to provide a more restful sleep, doesn't qualify as a "can't live without." Nor does a waterbed crib, whose major advantage seems to me to be that the bed is always warm. Despite testimonials in advertisements, there's no evidence that babies in waterbed cribs sleep better or have less colic.

Use your common sense when buying toys and equipment. If something looks like fun, makes your life a little easier, and you can afford it, enjoy it. But there is nothing among the myriad items at Baby Expos that is essential to a child's well-being.

CLOTHING FOR CHILDREN

One of my pet peeves is the tendency to dress children as minature adults. For a social gathering, one of my friends dressed her eighteen-month-old son in a child's version of a man's suit. After about five minutes, his tie was off, his shirttails were out of his pants, and his collar was askew. Little necks were not made for adult shirt collars. I think children should be allowed to remain children; they grow up soon enough.

Europeans seem to dress their children much more sensibly than Americans do. The typical European outfit for an infant or toddler is a one-piece knit garment, long-legged in the winter and short-legged in the summer, sometimes with a blouse or shirt underneath. This style of dressing appeals to me because the middle of the baby is covered and protected. Shirts don't pull out of pants, and the child looks neat. Moreover, the garment is flexible and expands with the child, fitting well through several size changes.

My favorite dress for American children is OshKosh B'gosh–type overalls with a shirt underneath. These overalls are loose and comfortable, will accommodate to a child's growth, and shirttails stay in. The current trend for designer children's clothes strikes me as silly. It wouldn't surprise me to see babies in Beverly Hills with red and green Gucci stripes on their diapers. While it may be fun for grandparents to give Pierre Cardin shirts, parents can be more sensible.

When children start to walk, I tell their parents to buy the least expensive tennis shoes they can find. It's not necessary to spend $30 or more on high-top special shoes for the beginning walker, no matter what the ads say. High-top shoes are designed for children whose heels don't protrude enough to hold a shoe. However, highly engineered, expensive shoes don't allow a toddler to flex the feet and toes and experience the ground. Since toddlers outgrow their shoes long before they wear them out, the most economical footgear is most practical.

I do confess to one personal weakness: I love patent-leather Mary Janes for little girls, and it seems to me that every little girl should have a pair for dress up.

ELEVEN

The Normal Stages of Development

STARTING in the 1950s and following their study population for thirty years, child psychiatrists Stella Chess and Alexander Thomas produced landmark research about early personality structure, reaching some fascinating and, I think, valid conclusions. According to Chess and Thomas, nine temperamental characteristics, which appear to be universal, determine the way a child reacts to the outside world and to parents. In addition to innate intelligence, these characteristics play an important role in the way a child develops.

The first category of temperament, *activity level,* is apparent from the moment a baby is born, and even *in utero.* An extremely active baby will be quicker to move around and roll over, sit up alone and walk. A more passive baby, the one who is content to lie in a crib examining the way fingers intertwine, will be slower to walk but quicker in mastering fine motor coordination, such as using two fingers to pick up small objects. The quiet baby will be slower in general than the active baby, which sometimes causes concern to parents. It shouldn't. Within the normal range, variations in development will have no relation to basic intelligence.

The second characteristic has to do with *regularity,* and refers to the child's internal clock. From the beginning, some babies are hungry every three hours and have a bowel movement twice a day at the same time every day. These children are likely to be easier to toilet train and will have fewer problems going to bed at the same time every night. Parents of the less regular child can't rely on scheduled times to play with their baby.

The third characteristic involves the way the child *responds to a new situation.* The child who is more cautious is likely to hang back, figure things out before exploring the world. These children are not inhibited. They look before they leap and may appear to be slower because they consolidate all their resources before taking a new step. A child like this may not walk until the age of fifteen months but may then master walking in one day. The child who approaches new situations more spontaneously, on the other hand, will reach for a new toy, try a new skill, taste a new food earlier and more easily than the cautious child.

The fourth trait, *adaptability to change in routine,* can be a positive characteristic if you have a flexible child. The child who has difficulty adapting to change will not flourish until the stress of a new situation subsides. Change can be anything from introducing a cup to giving up naps or going on vacation. The child who finds it difficult to adapt to new situations will find change difficult all through childhood. With this type of child, parents may have to be more flexible, making adjustments themselves while they are waiting for the child to adjust.

Chess and Thomas also describe differences in what they call *threshold of responsiveness,* or the degree of sensitivity to distractions and stimuli in the environment. A baby who can sleep in the midst of turbulence is not particularly sensitive to stimuli. A child who is easily awakened by noises or who cries upon hearing a harsh word will respond differently to later discipline and limitations. The sensitive child needs only to be told once not to touch the knobs on the stereo, while with the less responsive it may be necessary for a parent to repeat an admonition many times before eliciting the appropriate behavior. Again, this doesn't mean that the second child is more intelligent than the first, or vice versa.

Chess and Thomas also uncovered a variability in children's *basic moods.* Some children are happy and outgoing by nature; others are more serious and contemplative. What effect can this have on development? Smiles and laughs are the reward that adults receive when they play with or cuddle an infant. The child who smiles and laughs all the time may have the advantage of more social interaction and may, for example, talk earlier than the more introspective child.

Another difference between children relates to what Chess and Thomas call the *intensity of response.* For example, some children will respond to sensations of hunger or pain with piercing cries, while others may only whimper. For obvious reasons parents of intense children often respond quickly. Since these children are "rescued" immediately when they are in trouble, they may have less opportunity to try out solutions to situations and may not learn tasks and skills as quickly as the less intense child.

Another important characteristic is *distractibility.* The infant who is easily distracted by anything that moves or makes noise may take an hour for a feeding. The infant who sucks on a bottle or breast despite distractions will later be the child who can do homework in the middle of the living room with the TV on. In infancy this sort of child will attend to a task in spite of your best efforts at diversion. The easily distractible child probably will become the terror of the supermarket, and you might think twice before taking this child to a crowded restaurant.

The last personality trait is what is called *persistence,* or stick-to-it-iveness. Persistent children will not only stay with a task, despite repeated failure, until they achieve mastery, but they also may be in frequent conflict with parents by persisting until they get what they want. The less persistent child, with a shorter attention span, will give up easily if a task is frustrating and may take longer to learn complex tasks.

The variations just described all fall within the normal range of development, and there are no intrinsic gender differences. Boy babies are not on the whole more active than girl babies, and girl babies are not sweeter and gentler than boy babies. But through our own cues as parents, we tend, consciously or unconsciously, to reinforce the behaviors we define as "feminine" or "masculine." If a baby boy is vigorous and well coordinated, we reinforce the behavior by throwing balls and encouraging further athletic activity. By the same token, a girl is more often praised when she is quiet and gentle.

The most important thing here is that you express love for your child, that you share with your son or daughter the concept of the world as an interesting place, and that you encourage exploration of all the wonders to be seen and heard and touched and tasted. If you understand and accept your child's individual characteristics, you may be better able to understand the speed at which certain skills develop. You can then fashion your own approach to your own child.

We've already talked about the newborn in Chapter Two, so we'll start with the infant at one month old.

ONE TO THREE MONTHS

By this time, parents are more rested, schedules have been established, and everyone is settling into the household routine. The baby begins to show a different response to each parent: mother means eating and satisfying basic needs; father more often means play. The baby may become quiet and calm when mother approaches, but excited and smiling when father comes near. This is the beginning of one of the later great rewards of fatherhood: an excited chorus of "Daddy's home, Daddy's home!" at the end of the working day.

At this stage babies also become more interested in the world around them and may follow people and objects with their eyes, sometimes smiling spontaneously. They can chortle and squeal with delight, and make windmill-like movements with their arms and kick their legs. Babies who need the further comfort of sucking may use their thumbs or call on the middle two fingers. One small patient of mine favors her fourth finger with her hand backward, and another sucks only on her forearm. During this time, babies may suck as much as four hours a day, not because they're insecure, but as a way of exploring their bodies and discovering how to comfort themselves.

A baby exploring the body will concentrate on the interplay of fingers for many minutes. He or she may intertwine fingers and turn hands this way and that, regarding them as if they were toys.

Head control improves now. The head may still droop a little if you pull the baby up by the hands, but in general your baby is acquiring more stability and control. While lying face down, a baby will be able to lift the shoulders and part of the stomach as well as the head.

Chewing and drooling begin, but the baby isn't teething. Teeth may start erupting at four months, but some babies don't teethe until close to one year. Chewing as well as licking and putting things into the mouth are all ways for the baby to explore the environment.

By the age of two or three months, a baby may hold a rattle for a short time, then drop it and be surprised by its noise. If you remove objects from your baby's sight, no effort will be made to see where they went. This is in contrast to a few months from now, when babies learn that out of sight does not necessarily mean something is gone for good.

At this time, the baby may delightedly imitate sounds, the earliest stage of speech.

FOUR TO SIX MONTHS

This is my favorite baby age, although I love them all. Babies are not yet afraid of strangers and take delight in everything, laughing at the slightest provocation. Now (when colic usually subsides) is the time when parents often say, "So that's why I had a baby!"

The baby's head and back will be stronger, and some infants can sit unassisted by the fifth or sixth month. This leads to the discovery of the joy of independent movement.

It's too early for the baby to crawl; and, as we mentioned earlier, many babies never crawl, but scoot around on their stomachs to grab a toy that's out of reach.

Babies have been playing with their hands for quite some time now, but feet are new territory. Feet as well as anything else go directly into the mouth, and anything in reach is fair game to be felt, banged, rattled, mouthed, turned over, or thrown.

Babies can now recognize their names. They can roll back and forth from stomach to back although perhaps not yet from back to stomach, and some may propel themselves along the floor by rolling over. At a later creeping or crawling stage, many babies go backward at first; this seems to be easier than going forward. Some babies may have a slightly perplexed look on their faces before they figure out what's wrong. They will also experiment with sounds and produce wonderful noises on their own. In contrast to previous months, however, if you try to encourage your baby to imitate your sounds, the baby may withdraw and stop altogether.

Now that the child can manage an upright position some of the time, hands can be used separately and together. The child will use both hands to reach for an object and then transfer it from one hand to the other. This is when you must be careful about dangerous objects. A cup of hot liquid at the edge of a table is only one example.

As solid food is introduced, some children may want to hold the bottle themselves during a feeding.

Paper is a favorite texture to explore, and you may find yourself frequently extracting bits of paper from the baby's mouth. Be sure not to let the baby play with newspaper; the ink in newspaper print often contains lead.

This may be the appropriate time for a mother to return

to work. The baby isn't yet experiencing separation anxiety and isn't yet afraid of strangers.

At this stage, mirrors can be used to help the baby explore the boundaries of the body. Infants of four to six months laugh delightedly as they reach for the baby in the mirror and try to figure out how Mommy can be both behind and in front of the mirror.

The four to six month old loves to stand with feet flat, while an adult holds the trunk steady. This will not cause bowed legs, as was once believed. This reflex to push against a surface and use the legs for support, oddly enough, disappears at about seven or eight months and reappears when the child is ready to stand.

Playing peekaboo may send your six month old into rapturous giggles, and the baby will seem never to tire of the game. It usually starts with parents peeking from behind their hands, but babies rapidly learn to cover their faces with a blanket, then push it off. This is a developmental step on the road to trusting. It may also represent the baby's first "joke."

SEVEN TO NINE MONTHS

By now babies are able to pull themselves up on anything that promises to help them off the ground. Some placid babies may still be content merely to sit or lie and explore the world from narrower limits. If you have such a child, don't be concerned that your baby is slow; be happy you're not yet on the run throughout the house after your baby. A playpen gives the baby a safe area in which to begin to pull up, stand, and walk around while you're otherwise engaged.

Although some babies may now be able to stand, many aren't yet able to sit back down. They don't seem to have the ability to figure out how to bend in the middle, and you may find yourself coming to the aid of your standing baby many times during the day.

With all this newfound independence, feeding may become a problem. All of a sudden, the child doesn't want to take food from you but wants to play with it and eat only what happens to land in the mouth. A useful trick is to give the child small pieces of soft food to occupy both hands while you come down the middle with a spoon.

At this time a child may develop a fear of strangers. Forcing a child to accept strangers will be counterproductive and only make the problem worse. Remember that this is a normal developmental stage. Be patient, allowing your child to warm up to people at his or her own pace.

Nine month olds may crawl from one room to another, but invariably they will come back and look through the door to make sure you are still there. In a similar vein, a child will discover that calling "Mama" loudly from another room will bring Mommy and may try this many times a day.

Your neighbor's child may have started walking at nine months; but if your child hasn't, don't be discouraged. Most children don't start until twelve or fifteen months.

TEN TO TWELVE MONTHS

Now the baby is actively exploring, eager to pull up and move around. Your one year old may fall repeatedly, so expect bangs and bruises.

Various inexplicable fears may develop now and in the next year. There may be new fears or anxiety about familiar objects and people (such as the vacuum cleaner, strangers at the door, or even Grandma) that weren't formerly causes of concern. Periods of increasing independence and exploration seem to require a reversion to clinging and further reassurance. It's not useful at these times to push the child or dismiss these fears. With patience and reassurance, you will ultimately foster self-confidence, and the child will be less fearful of further independence.

Now your baby develops what is called a "pincer grasp," using the thumb and forefinger delicately to pick up all kinds of tiny objects, especially those on the floor. Since these may be things you don't want the baby to have, pay special attention to what may go into the baby's mouth.

This pincerlike movement allows the baby to eat small pieces of food such as Cheerios or soft cooked peas. I think the major function of Cheerios is to keep toddlers happy—at home and in their pediatrician's office.

During this time, a baby joyfully says "Mama" and "Dada," and can differentiate between the names for each parent. The child has already figured out that saying "Mama" brings Mommy, but for some unknown reasons many babies will now stop saying "Mama" and say "Dada" all the time. Although babies can wave "bye-bye" at this age, they often do it after the person has left the room. If so, you'll just have to wait until later to show off your baby's expertise.

Until now, most babies have been using either hand to reach for or grasp objects. At ten to twelve months, a child may reach with one hand more often than the other and transfer objects from the active to the passive hand in order to reach for something else.

For babies beginning to walk, days are exciting and tension-filled. After so much stimulation, many one year olds rock and bang their heads against their cribs at night. This behavior may seem odd, but it's only a means of self-comfort and tension release. Unfortunately the repeated banging may keep the household awake. The solution is to oil all the screws and joints on the crib and put a thick rug underneath to muffle the noise. The behavior itself, however, is as normal as thumb sucking and will eventually subside when it no longer serves a purpose. Although it may occasionally raise a bruise on the baby's forehead, head banging won't cause any damage to the brain or the shape of the skull.

Children may not know many actual words at this age, but they may identify pictures by saying "bowwow," for example, when they see a picture of a dog. Children also will imitate parents' activities, dusting the furniture with a diaper or trying to brush their own hair.

When your child starts to walk, you may notice the lack of an arch in the fat little foot and assume that your child has flat feet. Well, that's true. Children have a pad of fat on the bottom of the foot that makes the foot appear flat until about age five. The feet may turn in a little and the child may appear slightly bowlegged, but there is no need to worry. These transitory deformities are also normal.

TWELVE TO EIGHTEEN MONTHS

Everything accelerates now. Your baby will start to walk alone, and the experience is so filled with joy that many babies act giddy. In *The Magic Years,* Selma Fraiberg calls standing alone "a brave and lonely thing to do" and the mastery of walking "an exhilarating triumph." The child is demonstrating a new and an important motor skill, letting go of physical supports and, on a symbolic level, letting go of some emotional dependence. I love that first drunken-sailor type of walk with its broad-based gait for greater stability and the wad of diapers between the legs.

If your one year old is a quiet, self-contained baby, walking may not have the allure it holds for more vigorous children. One mother was disturbed when her daughter hadn't walked by fifteen months. I pointed out to her that not only were this child's other milestones in line, but her fine motor coordination was above-average. She was just a baby who was happy to study her toes or a single pea and had very little motivation for walking. She did start to walk shortly after she was fifteen months old.

There are families in which late walking is a familial characteristic. Fifty percent of late-walking children who are otherwise normal have a history of late walking in the family, compared with only 16 percent of children who walked earlier. If your otherwise normal child is a late walker, you may find a relative or two who also walked late.

At fifteen months, babies love to help with simple tasks. They are eager to participate in daily activities, and this is a lovely way to instruct your child about the routines. Savor this time when you can say "Put the diaper on the table," and your toddler will eagerly and smilingly perform the task. Remember this fifteen years from now when no amount of yelling or pleading can make your adolescent clean up that bedroom.

The independence that walking represents extends to other areas. The child may refuse to be fed by you and insist on making a mess while putting as little as possible into the mouth. If none of your tricks works, put a plastic sheet on the floor and accept the mess.

During this year, babies acquire an amazing number of words, increasing communication by leaps and bounds. An interesting thing about speech is that it must be learned from others. All the physical tasks that a normal child has previously mastered, such as using two fingers or walking, would have been learned anyway, but speech won't develop unless a child is spoken to and can hear what is being said. If, by the end of fifteen months, your child hasn't started saying a few words—only two or three besides "Mama" and "Dada" are enough—ask your pediatrician about testing your child's hearing. There may be nothing wrong—your child may not be programmed to speak until eighteen months—but the rare hearing problem can interfere with speech development. Obviously, the earlier problems are corrected, the better.

Television is not adequate stimulation for speech development. Acquisition of language requires active socializing with other humans. Television is a passive medium. Programs like "Sesame Street" are wonderful in their way and provide some stimulating material, but they are not a substitute for human beings. You can use programs like that only as an occasional and part-time baby-sitter for short periods of time. I would say half an hour is the limit.

At approximately eighteen months, children may start to put words together in their first sentences, although often the words they say are ones that only parents can understand. A child this age may say something in my office that sounds like a combination of Turkish and Hawaiian, and the mother will tell me it means "Cow pretty." I am amazed that children don't become more frustrated when they begin to talk. What they say seems of great importance to them, and no one can understand. After repeating these sentences many times, some give up, but they don't seem unduly upset.

During the early phases of language development, children can easily learn two languages at the same time. They also know the difference between the two, and can switch back and forth when talking to different people, often many times in one conversation. The programs that tout improved development for your child claim that you can teach a child a second language if you follow their program. The truth is, any child in a household where more than one language is spoken will learn the other language, and a child in a household where people don't regularly speak another language will not be bilingual to any useful extent.

I have a small patient, Leila, whose mother is Iranian and whose father is Japanese. Her parents met as students in Japan, where both spoke Japanese. Leila's mother's parents live with them and speak only Farsi. At home, mother and father speak Japanese to each other, but speak English outside the house. Leila knows all three languages and switches back and forth without any problem. Talk about a linguistic head start!

At about eighteen months, children also begin to interact socially with other children. This is the time that Mom-and-tot classes can be helpful not only for the mother, but also to give the child some experience with other children. If our urban society had evolved with better planning, we might have had common areas like the New England village green, where young and old could sit and visit while the children played together in everyone's view. Mom-and-tot classes are an attempt to re-create that sort of community.

At this age, children don't really regard other children as playmates. They play alongside each other, and the concept of sharing is entirely foreign. It's more common to grab something and yell "mine" than to play cooperatively.

Increased mobility in a curious toddler makes babyproofing your surroundings mandatory. Actually, there probably isn't anything that's truly babyproof except a padded room with bean-bag furniture, but see the discussion on safety in Chapter Nine for more specifics.

Some children can now remove a garment if given enough time and can help in dressing and undressing. Some of the babies who frequent my office and are no longer afraid of me may actually lift up their shirts when they see me coming with my stethoscope.

During the first half of this second year, toddlers learn to identify their body parts. They won't necessarily name them but can point to them when asked. A child's level of understanding at this age far exceeds the ability to talk, and you may be amazed by how much your toddler understands. One of my mothers told me that she asked her husband where a certain record album had gone, and her eighteen-month-old daughter went to get it.

Best of all, this is an age when you can start to ask for and receive hugs and kisses. Some babies never like to snuggle, some grow into it, and some are snugglers from the beginning. If you have the third type of child, count your blessings.

Walking is old hat by the end of this period, and your child won't be wobbling so much. Spills and bumps are just as frequent, however, because the toddler is starting to climb. Be sure there are gates on the stairs and that upstairs windows have grills. Also, if you have bookcases or furniture with lower drawers or shelves, anchor these to the wall. They can be toppled by a vigorous, climbing child.

EIGHTEEN TO TWENTY-FOUR MONTHS

Your baby is now adept at using a spoon and can self-feed with a minimum of mess. Simple articles of clothing can be put on and taken off alone. Children this age are beginning to stack blocks and build things. Taking small objects out of containers and putting them back can occupy a lot of time. Children begin to scribble with a pencil or crayon now.

Many children may become frustrated by the limitations parents impose, and temper tantrums may start.

Tantrums are the result of anger and frustration, and such

emotional outbursts should be tolerated to the extent we are able—we all feel angry or frustrated on occasion. If a tantrum distresses you and you try to stop it, not only are your attempts likely to be futile, but the child will realize that a tantrum can elicit a response. Any response, positive or negative, is a reinforcement. Let the temper tantrum run its course. Be sure the child can't come to any harm, then walk away a bit and wait for the outburst to end. Tantrums are usually a problem until well after the second birthday. It's difficult to let your child have a snit fit in the middle of the supermarket, but if you do it now, you may nip the problem in the bud. You might also examine whether your demands are too rigid or you're expecting too much of your child. See Chapter Twelve on discipline for more pointers about tantrums.

Your eighteen to twenty-four month old will name objects, identify animals in books, and can point to Mommy's nose as well as his or her own—a very important distinction to learn. Body balance is better, and the child can bend over and pick up an object, returning to an upright position without falling over.

Some children around the age of two may have a favorite object, usually a soft blanket, that they carry around constantly and cling to fondly, especially in times of stress. A child doesn't become attached to these objects because of insecurity; in fact, according to a study in the *Journal of the American Academy of Child Psychiatry,* half the children of normal I.Q. formed an attachment to an object in infancy. Few children with developmental disorders were attached to a treasured object. In other words, it's a normal for a child to form such an attachment. The transitional object, named thus because it eases a child's transition from dependence to independence, allows the child to take along a familiar object that gives a sense of home and self to the unfamiliar and sometimes frightening outside world.

Toddlers need periods of unbridled freedom, and the wide open spaces of a park or playground offer important opportunities for freedom of movement not available at home. Visit the park as often as possible, and keep a loose rein on your child.

THE TWO YEAR OLD

By the end of this year, your child may start to recognize colors, say his or her own name, first and last, and draw circles instead of aimless scribbles.

Younger children can only understand one thing at a time, but a two year old can grasp concepts like "yesterday," "later," and "tomorrow." Two year olds are just starting to understand the difference between "real" and "pretend." Also, the idea that there is a life in the mind, that thinking can be directed, develops. One of the nurses in my office remembers when her daughter was close to three. As they were riding in the car, the child said, "Mommy, I'm talking, and you can't hear me!" With great delight, the child understood that she was thinking.

We've all heard about the "terrible twos," but, there are "terrific twos." Some children never exhibit the famous rebellion of the two year old, and some postpone this period until they are three or four.

However, two year olds are mostly in perpetual motion. Parents often ask me if their child is hyperactive, but usually the child is just a normal two year old. As a pediatrician, I can say that the two year olds are difficult to examine medically. They'll sit and talk to me very pleasantly for several minutes but turn into whirling and dervishes as I approach to examine them. Fine motor coordination has become more sophisticated; for the two year old, turning knobs and removing jar tops present no difficulty. This is the peak age for accidental poisoning. So be sure you have some ipecac on hand and know how to use it. See also Chapter Nine on safety.

As part of an on-going experiment in how much control a child can exert over the world, your child may want to have a voice in some decisions. You should be indulgent, for a child is learning the roots of self-care and decision making. If you ask the child to make a decision or to give an opinion, however, you must be prepared to accept it. I make this mistake occasionally in my office. I *should* say, "Now I'm going to listen to your chest," but I forget and say, "May I listen to your chest?" The answer is invariably "No," and then what can I do? You might ask your child if he or she wants to wear the blue shirt or the brown shirt, but don't ask your child if he or she wants to go to bed. That's not his or her decision.

Having decided to give a child some voice in decision making, prepare yourself to live by it, even if the decision is not exactly to your liking. One of the nurses in my office was in a children's store and overheard the following conversation: A mother and her two-year-old daughter were shopping for a dress for the child. The mother preferred the blue dress, and the child wanted the pink one. The mother finally said, "But, dear, you look so pretty in the blue dress. It matches your eyes."

As the mother turned away to pay for the blue dress, the little girl sighed dramatically and said out loud but to herself, "I wish I had pink eyes."

One of the most difficult judgments parents must make as their children grow up is how much to intervene and how much to hang back. By allowing your child the physical and emotional space to explore the world at whatever pace feels best, you will enhance your child's developmental potential without creating stress to perform. If learning ABC's is fun for both of you, by all means teach the alphabet to your child and praise the accomplishment. But if your child would rather climb into an empty cardboard carton to play train, that's just as valuable as learning the alphabet.

TOILET TRAINING

When your child is close to two years old, friends and relatives will expect you to toilet train. I say "expect" because people often imply that something is wrong with children or parents if the child is not trained by the age of two. There is no correlation between a child's intelligence or the quality of parenting and the age at which toilet training succeeds. Toilet training should be relaxed and easy. The child will master it sooner or later, and anytime that the child is ready is all right. Two is only the average age at which *some* children are ready to be trained and the age at which I advise my patients to begin training. Some children may master it earlier, and many are neither ready nor interested until age three or older.

There is only one reason why a child would be interested in using a toilet—parental approval. There are a few children who express discomfort when their diapers are wet, and these may be easier to train, but urine and stool are not repugnant to children. On the contrary, stool is perceived as a part of their bodies. This is reinforced when a parent shows approval and happiness when a child leaves a stool for them in a potty chair or in a toilet. But then this valued gift is flushed away. Is this any way to treat an object of value? It makes no sense to children.

Therefore, the only way to enlist the cooperation of a two

year old in what seems to them a silly endeavor is to offer approval. The child's subsequent feeling of accomplishment at mastering what parents want and appear to expect will keep the toddler using the pot.

I tell parents to do as little as possible about toilet training before age two. Keep a potty chair next to the toilet from the time the child is eighteen or twenty months old. The toilet itself is difficult for the child to climb onto, and toileting is more comfortable if the feet can rest on the floor. Also, the child doesn't have direct contact with that big machine that can be a source of fear, with its swirling, roaring water that sucks things away into its depths. The child may want to help flush when parents use the toilet, and familiarity with the noise and swirling water may help to diminish that fear. Seeing Mom and Dad use the toilet may prompt the child to imitate sitting on the potty, for which you should give approval.

When parents use the toilet, explain from time to time what you are doing. Choose the words you want to use for these bodily functions. I don't think there's anything wrong with saying "potty" or "tinkle," but decide on a consistent term. If you want to say "urinate" or "defecate," fine. But the child who said to me "I have to micturate" was asked to be a little too clinical, I thought.

After deciding what you're going to call urine and stool, say in a matter-of-fact way, "I see you're wet. Let's change your diaper," or "Oh, you've made a do-do. Let's clean you up." After that, associate the act with the place to do it. If your child needs to have a diaper changed, put the child on the potty for a few minutes while you tend to the soiled diaper. If your toddler seems to be in the process of having a stool, gently guide the child to the potty, not necessarily taking the diapers down before the act is over.

If your child regularly produces a BM at the same time each day, you may anticipate the act. Remain close to the potty at that time, and place the child on it when you see it begin. But always remember that each stool is not a pivotal event. A frantic spurt of activity to race to the potty chair may only engender anxiety about reaching the potty in time and may create rather than solve problems.

Before a child can be trained, there are several prerequisites. A child who sucks on a bottle all day urinates so frequently that to attempt toilet training would be silly. You must wait until the child is dry for several hours at a time. The child also must be able to follow simple commands such as "Pull up your pants" and "Open and close the lid of the potty chair."

If a child happens to produce urine or stool while sitting on the potty chair, show that you are pleased and interested, but never, never punish a child for not producing. Avoid pressure or shame, and accept this as a process that may take quite a while, with periods of regression or disinterest as a natural part of the plan. During a bout of illness, for example, toilet training may be forgotten, and rightly so. Express no anger or dissatisfaction over a temporary failure, for a child will be feeling bad enough at those times.

When your child seems interested and ready, use training pants that are a little too big, so the child can easily pull them up or down. If clothing takes too long to maneuver, the child won't make it to the potty chair in time no matter how good the intentions. For this reason, many people postpone toilet training until the warmer months of the year, when a child has less clothing with which to contend.

Some books tell you not to read to a child during training because it gives a false notion of the potty's purpose. But this may be futile advice. One of the nurses in my office told me that her little girl would never go to the potty without a newspaper or magazine. Of course, she couldn't read and as often as not held the material upside down. But everyone else in the house read while they were in the bathroom, and she was not about to be left out.

A doll that wets may be useful to teach a child the steps necessary for independent toileting. Dress the doll in diapers or training pants. Teach the child the difference between wet and dry. Give the doll a drink and demonstrate the connection between wet diapers and water coming from the doll. You can teach the child to take the doll through the steps from going to the potty, lowering pants or diapers, sitting on the potty, waiting for urine, wiping, and pulling up the pants. Also, praise the doll for being dry and for producing in the potty.

This doll play should only be done when the child is interested and should only last as long as you're both enjoying it. That may be for five minutes or for an hour, depending on your child's mood and how entertaining you make it.

Rewarding desired behavior with approval—a hug, a smile—is always the most effective way to encourage certain behaviors in children. When your child uses the toilet and when diapers or pants are dry, give the child praise. Daytime dryness is the first goal, but nighttime dryness has to occur in its own time.

Small children are almost never dry through the night. In fact, it's normal for some children not to achieve nighttime dryness until age six or later. You may have to use a diaper for naps and bedtime for a few years, even though your child is dry during the day. A developmental lag between daytime dryness and nighttime wetness is normal, and a child can have very little control over it. If there's a history of bedwetting at later ages in the mother or father, the child may continue to wet the bed until the age at which the parent stopped. Isn't that an interesting phenomenon? I can't imagine how something like that can be programmed.

When you're toilet training, remember that all you're doing is encouraging a behavior that is inevitable sooner or later. Your child walked when the time was right, started using words when the time was right, and will use the toilet when the time is right.

TWELVE

Discipline: Training Your Child the Woodhouse Way

ONE OF MY PATIENTS had been having problems in her marriage. When she came to me recently, I asked how things were going. "Much better," she said.

I asked her what made the difference.

"I read a book about training your dog by Barbara Woodhouse. I applied some of her principles to my relationship with my husband, and they worked," she said, adding, "don't ever tell him that!"

I called this chapter "Training Your Child the Woodhouse Way" not because I believe in using a metal choke chain on children, but because the Woodhouse approach of clear, appropriate expectations, simple and easily understandable commands, rewards, praise, and mutual respect apply equally to children and dogs. Woodhouse stresses encouraging acceptable behavior while keeping in mind that the dog and master should enjoy their relationship, as I've emphasized for parents and children throughout this book.

Strong, clear discipline is as important to a child's development as freedom is. The optimal environment strikes a balance between freedom to further a child's intellectual development and satisfy curiosity, and enough restraint for physical safety.

EDUCATION AND PROTECTION

When adults think of discipline, punishment most often comes to mind. But discipline really means education and protection, education in socially acceptable behavior and protection from indulging in potentially dangerous behavior. More than just setting rules and dispensing punishment, discipline imparts values, an attitude toward life and how to live it with others. If discipline is to serve its purpose, the child should develop a sense of confidence and self-respect that lasts a lifetime. Since we're dealing here with the child through age two, protection from harm and an introduction to socially acceptable behavior are the primary orientation of discipline. There is no such thing as a conscience in a child under two: the issue of right and wrong depends entirely on parental approval and disapproval. Parents often tell me that their eighteen month old stands in front of a forbidden cabinet saying "No, no" over and over, controlling his own behavior with his parents' words.

The object of discipline as education and protection is to create an environment with clear-cut, consistent boundaries within which the child can explore and develop safely and happily. If children feel secure and trusting, it's not uncommon for them to behave beautifully at other people's homes or at nursery school but to test the limits regularly at home. Many mothers tell me that the sitter or preschool teacher thinks the child is perfect. But then the mother sighs, "If only they knew how she acts at home." This apparently contradictory behavior is normal. Your child is testing the limits at home, where it's your job to set them.

Think of this behavior like a dog chasing a car. The dog doesn't really want to catch the car—he wouldn't know what to do with it if he did. The child doesn't really want unbridled freedom—it would be too much to handle. If, as parents, you have given your child secure boundaries and consistent limitations, your child can safely challenge these at home.

When parents create an atmosphere of trust and consistency, the child understands limitations and expectations. Parents benefit too: they can relax and enjoy their children.

Several factors affect discipline styles: the personality of the parents; the mother's and father's own parents, whom they may be unconsciously reacting against or imitating; the degree to which parents agree with each other on discipline; and the personality of the child.

Parents model their parenting behavior after their own parents. A person who was raised in a highly controlled environment will most likely have difficulty with a loose, tumultuous household. Parents who had what they perceive as overbearing, rigid parents may react by being extravagantly permissive with their children.

In *The Magic Years,* Selma Fraiberg compares toddler discipline to the arrival of the missionaries among the natives. The joyful savage has been swinging freely through the jungle and must now observe restrictions that seem to make no sense. All of a sudden the child is told there are some things that can be touched and others that cannot be touched, and, to an innocent child, there's no rhyme or reason to it. If we accept that this makes no sense to a child, we can see that at least we must be consistent about the rules.

But don't be surprised if you find difficulty in being consistent. You may have arose from the wrong side of the bed and had a twelve-hour day of minor annoyances. Your daughter then commits a minor misdemeanor such as picking her nose, and you suddenly fly into a rage. You're being inconsistent, but you're also being human. All the discussions you hear and read, including this one, mention consistency over and over, but this really refers to basic major issues. All human beings are inconsistent—parents most of all. Just be aware of your goals, and try your best daily. As long as you're *usually* consistent, the sum of days, weeks, and months will add up to enough consistency.

You and your partner must also agree on what you find acceptable before you try to impose these limitations on your child. Often, two parents have disparate styles of discipline, based on different backgrounds. Different styles can be effective together as long as you agree on the fundamental issues. If the refrigerator door is considered off-limits by one parent, it must also be considered off-limits by the other. If one parent prohibits ball throwing in the house, so must the other.

Not to agree will confuse your child. Rebecca's parents never agreed on what to do when she wakes up at night. (This is only the tip of the iceberg, for they have conflict in other areas of their lives together.) When Rebecca awakens, one parent wants to put her back into her bed while the other wants to take her into their bed. The issue is not who's right or wrong—there is almost never an absolute right or wrong in situations like these. What's important is that the couple decide on a course of action and pursue it consistently. By arguing over it, they're just prolonging the conflict and their daughter's sleeplessness. I thought it might be better to let her sleep with one or both parents, but I really didn't care as much about that as the fact that they should agree about what to do.

Parents should respect their children, just as children need to respect their parents. Recently, while talking to a mother about her infant, her two-year-old son predictably and understandably tried to interrupt our conversation, for we hadn't been paying attention to him for quite a while. She slapped him noisily on the side of the face and said, "Shut up!" Not only is a slap on the face never acceptable—for it could be physically harmful—but it's demeaning to the child. It doesn't teach him what would be acceptable so that he can alter his behavior but only says that he is a "bad boy."

If the mother is annoyed by her son's interruption, it would be more instructive and more respectful to tell him, in a firm tone of voice, that he must wait until she had finished speaking before he can talk. Parents who treat their children with respect also reward their children with a hug, a smile, a word of praise when acceptable behavior reigns, and don't shame or degrade them when a mistake is made. This doesn't mean, however, that parents aren't allowed to be angry.

Some people feel that they may have failed as parents if they blow up over their children's behavior. A parent is human, and a child's behavior may trigger reactions affected by the parent's own state of mind. A mother may recognize traits in her child that she wishes she didn't have herself. Dissatisfaction with herself may trigger excessive anger at similar behaviors in her child. Unresolved anger toward a parent's sibling may be expressed toward a child whose behavior rouses feelings of frustration reminiscent of the earlier relationship.

Also, parents deal with their own day-to-day stresses, and children are handy targets upon which parents may vent their feelings. If marital or financial stress causes parents to feel anxious or helpless, their children may become the target of their frustrated feelings. See the story of David later in this chapter.

There is nothing wrong if parents lose their tempers with children. Just as we must allow children to vent their feelings, so must parents be allowed this privilege. However, as an adult, try to take a moment to examine how appropriate your anger is and whether it's directed at the right target. Are you really blowing up because of the child, or is something else bothering you and making you short-tempered? It's understandable for a parent to feel frustrated with a baby whose colic causes ceaseless crying, but to express that as anger toward the infant is inappropriate. If you find yourself angry at your infant, decompress, and give yourself a respite from the constant crying by taking a shower or a walk around the block. Turn the baby over to the other parent or to a neighbor until you regain perspective.

Sometimes a parent who blows up at a toddler in the evening realizes that the child has been asking for discipline in many small ways all day. The "bad day" that many two year olds and their mothers have results from minor misbehaviors that have piled up until mother is angry enough to lower the boom. Perhaps a little boom lowering earlier in the day might have saved them both from several hours of increasing tension. Remember that children need those limits, and be alert to children's subtle demands for control.

If a parent feels a strong, physical rage—and almost all parents have times when they would like to let loose physically—banging a rolled-up newspaper on a table top makes a satisfying sound and alerts the child that you've reached your tolerance limit. Or beat a belt on a chair. Never hit your child out of anger. Take five or ten breaths before you vent your feelings physically. If you must rid yourself of the discomfort generated by strong feelings, tear up your bed and pound the pillows, throw dirty diapers out of the window, sit down and cry—do anything physically safe that makes you feel better. If you worry that you may actually physically harm your child, talk to someone right away. If your spouse isn't available or sympathetic, call your pediatrician or even a child-abuse hotline before raising your hand to your child. Feelings must find expression, and children who see their parents venting their feelings in safe ways learn that it's normal to have strong feelings and that there are acceptable ways to release them.

A child's own personality will also determine how easily a parent can educate and protect. The quiet child who is content to contemplate his fingers for hours on end will need less intervention than the active child who pokes and prods, explores and climbs continuously. The persistent child who doggedly pursues a goal despite obstacles will be harder to divert or control than one who is less persistent.

One-year-old Lisa was always an easy child. If her gentle, reserved mother said "No" firmly, Lisa would stick out her lower lip, stop what she was doing, and turn to something else. Her brother, Michael, was what Dr. Spock calls a "sparkler." As a toddler, nothing his mother did could deter him from his self-appointed tasks. When, in anger and frustration, she uncharacteristically spanked him on his diapered bottom, he turned around and hit her in return. Obviously, this mother had to develop different techniques for Michael and Lisa.

APPROPRIATE EXPECTATIONS FOR INFANTS

The concept of clear and appropriate expectations à la Barbara Woodhouse musts be based on a rational understanding of a child's abilities and needs at different ages. During the first months of a child's life, the concept of discipline is irrelevant. The demands of a small baby are an urgent call for needs to be met, and depriving an infant of your love and attention is never appropriate. Some people feel that babies have to be "disciplined" not to make frequent demands on their parents when they're not hungry or wet, and that if parents pick up a baby too often or respond to a cry for attention, they'll spoil the child.

On the contrary, a study at McGill University showed that infants who were carried not only when they were hungry or when they asked for comfort, but also at other times when they didn't seem to be demanding it, cried less overall than babies who were only picked up when they cried. Other similar studies have followed children for several years, and have shown that, far from spoiling a baby and creating a more demanding child, indulging and even overindulging an infant's need for contact will produce an ultimately happier and less demanding person. In other words, when your infant cries, follow your heart and pick the baby up whenever you can. The more comfort you give, the more secure your baby will be.

As a child begins to teethe, a breast-feeding baby may bite a mother's nipple. When nursing mothers ask me what to do, the answer is simple: all that's necessary is a sharp cry of pain, a loud "No," and removing the baby briefly from the breast. This cry startles the infant and makes the baby aware of your displeasure. The only times I've seen infants persist in biting their mothers' nipples were instances where babies were ready to be weaned anyway.

ANGER AND TANTRUMS

When children become mobile, toward the end of the first year, their world becomes both wider and narrower—wider because the child can explore beyond the limits of the crib or a parent's arms, and narrower because parents are constantly placing limits on exploration. The child is allowed to climb from the floor to the couch, so why not from the floor to the chair to the top of the stove? The child can reach in the toy box to remove an attractive toy, so why is that interesting glass in the dishwasher off limits? It's not surprising that "No" is the first clear word we hear from toddlers since they hear it so often from parents.

It's unrealistic to expect children under two to respect physical limitations, so minimize the amount of hazardous or forbidden material that's easy to reach. There will always be stereo knobs and television controls within reach, however, no matter what you do. A firm "No" is all that's necessary. If a second, sterner warning doesn't work, remove the child from the temptation and offer another diversion.

Toward the end of the first year, the ambitions of toddlers exceed their capabilities and their permitted boundaries, and frustration can cause tantrums and misbehaviors. I've often watched toddlers reaching into the cabinet under the sink in my examining room and attempting to slip their hands into the small space provided by the childproof locks. Some children stop shortly after they're thwarted, some persist until their hands are stuck, and others scream and bang on the door in rage. The last type of child needs to be diverted to another activity or helped to accomplish a task before frustration produces a tantrum.

If you give a child an acceptable alternative, you are issuing clear and understandable commands. Just saying "Don't make a mess" means little to a toddler drenching counter and clothes at a sink. If you turn the faucet to create a more manageable stream and show the child how to handle soap, you may avoid a tantrum while you teach the child an alternate acceptable behavior.

At first, children don't initiate tantrums just to manipulate parents. However, when tantrums elicit responses, they are reinforced. If you can't divert a tantrum, just make sure that the child can't be hurt and turn away until it's over. Recognize that a tantrum is an expression of anger and frustration. We all have snit fits when we're upset, and children should be allowed to blow off these feelings. Ignoring tantrums won't make them stop sooner, but interacting can prolong them.

Eighteen-month-old Billy had the worst case of tantrums I've ever seen. The first time I saw him he was taking anticonvulsant medications. His brain-wave tests and neurological examination were normal, but he had brief episodes of turning blue and twitching several times a day. Another doctor diagnosed them as seizures, but they were not controlled by medication. When Billy had one of his "seizures" in my office, the truth became plain: he was having tantrums with a "breath-holding spell," in which children who are hurt or angry suddenly let out a long cry, turn pale or blue, and then faint for a moment before they breathe again, sometimes twitching a little in the process. We suddenly realized that Billy's "seizures" always occurred when he was angry. He would throw himself on the floor in a tantrum, then have a breath-holding spell, turn blue, and twitch.

His tantrums were effective: his mother tried to do all she could to avoid upsetting him and precipitating these frightening episodes. Since there are no side-effects (except for maternal anxiety) to a breath-holding spell, we stopped the useless medication and let him have his tantrums. When his mother ignored them, Billy's tantrums became less frequent and less severe, and finally stopped. Since Billy could no longer control his mother through fear of a "seizure," there was little reward for his tantrums. The problem his mother had to deal with for a while was the appalled look on other people's faces when her son would throw himself on the ground, turn blue, have what appeared to be a seizure, and she would look on with calm indifference.

The message that children should receive is that tantrums don't accomplish or change anything. They may be necessary for blowing off steam, but they don't change "No" to "Yes." One of my mothers pretends her child is invisible until the tantrum simmers down. A mother who matter-of-factly acknowledges a child's tantrum and says "I'll talk to you when you're done" or who ignores it and continues whatever she was doing until the snit fit is over is telling the child that expressing strong feelings is all right, but a tantrum won't solve anything.

The toddler who bites another child is usually not doing so out of anger, but rather as a means of exploration, feeling, and testing as the child would feel and explore a toy with the mouth as well as with hands and eyes. Toddler biting is spontaneous and a surprise to the victim, for it doesn't arise out of conflict.

Biting will stop if the child is punished immediately. If the toddler bites a child who is more aggressive, larger, and stronger, that may be the end of biting, for the larger child may pack a significant wallop. If the child who is bitten is quiet and passive, the bites may go undetected until the playmate's mother discovers the marks at home. Then the punishment will not be connected to the crime, and discipline will not make any sense to the biter.

Many people think that an adult should bite the child back. On the surface that seems to make sense, but not if you think about it for a moment. If we are teaching a child that a behavior is unacceptable, how do we demonstrate that by performing the act ourselves? Also, adults must never bite hard enough to hurt, for that would rightly be considered a form of child abuse, harmful as well as inappropriate.

We want the child to understand that biting means that you will not be accepted, that you won't be allowed to live and play with others. It's inappropriate behavior. The point is best learned when an adult reacts to the child's behavior immediately after the act has taken place, so that the child can connect the punishment with the crime. State firmly and definitely that what the child did was unacceptable. Then, remove the child from the social situation for a short period of time, perhaps one or two minutes at first. Every time biting occurs after that, follow the same procedure, and increase the periods of isolation by one minute at a time. To a child this is a long time to be deprived of company. You can either seat the child in the corner like Dennis the Menace, isolate the biter in the laundry room, or use another safe place where you can observe the child while avoiding direct contact with others.

If that doesn't work and you're the sort of parent who can mete out physical punishment comfortably, a light slap on the hand or a "potch" on the bottom, as my family used to call it, may be effective. What's important for parents to remember is that a toddler who bites isn't mean, aggressive, or antisocial. Children merely experiment with many behaviors in their repertoire, and it's your job to communicate that nothing good happens when you bite.

THE TWO YEAR OLD AS TESTER

Two year olds are beginning to test the limits of their control over the world. Many two year olds answer "No" to everything, and books sometimes call this a negativistic age. However, "No" used by a two year old doesn't always mean "No"; it may just be a way to see what happens when you don't give consent to adult requests. After all, from a child's point of view, parents control children by using "No," so why shouldn't a child try it, too?

If your child is going through this "No" stage, avoid too many choices. Say "Now you're going to bed" rather than "Will you go to bed?" or "Would you like to hear another story and then go to bed?" so the child has less chance to try "No." By the same token, when the two year old tries to exert control by refusing to wear what you select, narrow the decision to two choices: "Do you want the brown shirt or the red shirt?" This allows the child to exercise some control without fostering conflict or confusion by offering too many choices.

You may now encounter occasions when physical punishment seems necessary, but I think this should be limited to life-threatening situations. If your child runs into the street or plays with the stove, a swat on a diapered bottom or a tap on the hands is acceptable and may communicate the gravity of the situation if physical means are not a usual form of discipline.

Two year olds need wide open spaces, frequent visits to playgrounds and parks, and the freedom to explore tirelessly in a safe environment.

I remember the case of two-year-old David and his mother, who had the most inappropriate expectations I've ever seen. The mother was referred by an orthopedist, whom she had consulted for her own back pain. No wonder she had back pain—David was a huge two year old, and carrying him around had taken its toll on her forty-year-old back. She mentioned to the orthopedist that David's pediatrician thought he was hyperactive and wanted to prescribe Ritalin, a stimulant commonly prescribed for hyperactive children but rarely at this young age. This didn't seem right to my orthopedic colleague, so he asked her to see me for another opinion.

When they arrived, I noticed that David was in a leash apparatus, although his mother removed it in the examining room. While we were talking, she constantly pulled him away from the trash can and examining table, and tried to make him sit still. Nothing in my office can harm children unless they climb on the sink and dive off head first, so I suggested she leave him alone while we talked. He went to the trash can and played with the revolving lid for a few minutes, then climbed on a small chair to reach the light switch. As we continued to talk, I told his mother not to move. Soon David lost interest in the gadgets in the room and started playing quietly with a puzzle on the floor.

David's mother and I discussed why she felt she had to control his behavior so closely. After all, a two year old is naturally active, I pointed out, and needs to touch, feel, and experiment with the world. She revealed that she had left family and friends in another state and felt alone and not in control of her life. She had no one to talk to, and her husband was wrapped up in his new job. Since David spent a lot of energy resisting his mother's excessive restrictions, he seemed hyperactive to her.

The truth is, David was a normal two year old whose mother had unrealistic expectations and, therefore, considered him a discipline problem. His mother was so unhappy herself that I recommended her to a counselor whom she is seeing. Now that she has someone in whom she can confide and work through her problems, and now that she can see that her expectations for her son were unrealistic, the situation seems to be improving.

While David's case is extreme, it illustrates that our expectations must be appropriate for a child's age and the fact that a parent's own emotional state determines the ease or difficulty of discipline. Children are exquisitely sensitive to their parents' moods, and misbehavior can sometimes be traced to the emotional climate at home. I'm not saying that you shouldn't try to restrict your child's behavior, but be aware of the times when your child may be responding to something in your life.

Parents feel that they are responsible for their children's behavior, and if, for example, a child is disruptive in public, they think they'll be regarded as poor parents. Also, when a child is being difficult, a parent's sense of control is threatened. But just as you allow your children to make mistakes and to learn from them, you must allow yourself to make mistakes as a parent. You're only human. If you feel you've flown off the handle inappropriately or done or said something you wish you hadn't, the best thing you can do is to apologize to your child. Far from weakening your position as a parent, your child learns that you are fair, that words are not immutable, that saying something does not write it in stone, and that relationships are based on honesty and clear understandings.

You can relax and enjoy your child when you accept the fact that you will be imperfect and inconsistent at times and that your child will have difficult moments, but that your overriding goal is to create an atmosphere at home of trust, mutual respect, and clear limitations.

THIRTEEN

Working Mothers: Wonder Woman Doesn't Exist

SALLY HAS FOUR CHILDREN. When the first two were born, Sally devoted herself to child rearing while her husband finished his education and launched his career. Now, at forty, with two younger children, Sally is a successful film editor. She and her husband share child care and home obligations. Sally's first two children were infants in the late 1960s; the second two were born in the 1980s. While Sally's situation may not be typical of family planning, her choices do reflect how career and family options have changed.

In 1982, half of all children under the age of six and 60 percent of those from six to sixteen had mothers who worked outside the home. Between 1972 and 1982, the number of women with professional degrees had increased 50 percent, and a great many of these women have postponed childbearing until they are well into their thirties.

From a child's point of view, the best of all possible worlds would be to have a stay-at-home mother. However, I would never argue that this is the best of all possible worlds for mothers and that they should leave the business world to men.

The reasons why women need to work or need to return to work are all too familiar. Financial necessity is the prime reason. Many families today cannot make ends meet without two paychecks. A single parent (and nine out of ten single parents are women) often has no choice. Women with careers may jeopardize their chances for advancement if they leave the work arena for a year or two. The same is true for entrepreneurs. Still other women need to work for self-fulfillment. And there's a last group: some mothers simply require the outside stimulus, at least on a part-time basis. The job itself may not be all-important; it's the change of scene that counts.

While I support and understand all these reasons for wanting to work, it seems to me that mothers (and fathers) sometimes confuse a higher standard of living with financial necessity. I'm distressed when I see couples give top priority to material things—when a mother's paycheck goes to pay for the recreational vehicle or a VCR, not what I would call necessities of life. If your main motive for returning to work is indulging in the "extras," consider whether you really want to be separated from your child during those precious first years. Could you manage almost as well with a lower standard of living for a few years? Unless the pay is extraordinarily good, by the time you add up the cost of day care, clothes, transportation, a possible change in tax bracket, plus the emotional cost to you and the reduced time you and your mate will have as a couple and as parents, you may find that working is not the best choice.

Part-time work to meet a specific expense is one compromise. One of my patients works part-time so her family can qualify for health insurance. Her husband is self-employed, and health insurance is prohibitively expensive for the small businessperson. By working for a supermarket chain for a minimum number of hours a week while her husband takes responsibility for child care, this woman provides health insurance for the whole family.

On the plus side, many husbands and wives with dual careers have a more stimulating relationship. Surveys indicate that women who are employed outside the home do feel greater satisfaction in their marriages. Also, a woman earning an income has a greater sense of self-worth and a feeling of control over her life. The argument can also be made that the woman who spends her working day with adults may be more captivated by a child when evening comes and may also have more energy than if she had been on hand for twenty-four hours.

The decision of when to return to work is an individual matter, depending on your feelings and those of your partner, your health, practical and financial considerations, the company policy where you work, and the child-care resources available to you. Probably the best time to get back to work is when your baby is between six and twelve weeks old. That's when most of my patients choose to return. The developmental fear of strangers hasn't occurred yet in infants of this age.

MAKE WORKING WORK FOR YOU

Wonder Woman doesn't exist; a working mother will have to make some compromises. One of my patients, a classical singer and master voice teacher, has reared two of the most psychologically intact, delightful sons I know. Some years ago I asked Bunny how she managed to cope with her myriad responsibilities. She told me that she realized early on that something had to give. With a husband, a career, two bright children who needed attention, and a house to manage, she couldn't be perfect on all counts. She decided that the house was the least important. Essentially, she gave up housekeeping, and, as I can attest, the house was a shambles—full of love, but a shambles.

My advice to women who work is always to let the house go to hell if you have to make a choice. Make whatever concessions you can with your partner to save time and energy. Giving full attention to your loved ones when they need it is more important than vacuuming the rug or having dinner parties.

You'll also be a better (and happier) wife and mother if you indulge yourself a little. Set aside some time for doing nothing. That's right, nothing—a time when you can just unwind and forget about all the things that need to be done. The things that need to be done will wait until you get to them, but a frayed temper or harried spirit will take the fun out of any family activity.

If you feel the need to decompress, take fifteen minutes after work and sit on a park bench or go window shopping. One of my colleagues plans to arrive fifteen minutes early to pick up her daughter from school. She leans back in her car, closes her eyes and meditates, takes a short nap, or just enjoys looking at the grass. She loves her fifteen-minute interlude and feels that it refreshes her and keeps her functioning well for the rest of the day.

Another woman, the mother of three and also a doctor, rises half an hour before the rest of the household. She either rides her bike or jogs around her neighborhood at dawn. Not only is she revitalized by the exercise, but she treasures this time. Sometimes she plans her day, and sometimes she lets her mind run free. Most important, she has a special half-hour alone for herself. This woman has also established a Saturday-night bath ritual. Yes, she bathes on other days, but on Saturday evening she takes a luxurious bubble bath. If she's on call, she asks the answering service to hold all but emergency calls for thirty minutes. During this time, her husband takes over with the children.

Still another working mother sets aside at least half an hour for personal reading before going to sleep. Sometimes she falls asleep with the book in her hand, but at least she can look forward each night to this private time.

No matter how liberated or enlightened men have become, it's still primarily the woman's responsibility to organize the household. Most men these days are willing, when asked, to share in household duties, but we still have a long way to go. Nevertheless, I sometimes hear of special acts of kindness and love that couples develop to care for each other and lighten the load.

While one of my patients takes her morning shower, her husband warms her towels in the dryer and removes them when he hears her shut off the shower. How frazzled can you be when your husband hands you warm towels as you step out of the shower?

You can create your own ways to find time for yourself. If you commute, whether you're in your own car with a tape deck or on public-transportation with a Walkman, you can play tapes of your favorite music or books. I've asked working mothers what they're doing for themselves, and I've found that half of them don't think of these small but important indulgences, and take no such time. I wish they would.

I know of one mother who still has a long drive after she picks up her son at the day-care center. After a pressured day, she often feels enervated and unable to join in when her bouncy son wants to sing and play in his car seat. She made a tape of herself singing all the verses to "Old MacDonald" and "Farmer in the Dell" and the child's favorites. On the drive home, the little boy sings along merrily with his mother on tape.

We've all heard a lot about "quality time" and how it is more important than the actual hours spent with a child. However, the concept of quality time can be stretched to a point where it becomes ridiculous. "Quality time" should not be confused with "make nice time," when a parent makes up for absence earlier in the day. It does mean time spent together in the daily activities of a household. Every moment with a child does not have to involve an "enriching" experience. And parents should feel able to converse between themselves without focusing all their attention on a child. So long as the child is playing companionably nearby and seems content, you can rest assured that all is well. It's the total family atmosphere that counts most.

DAY CARE: WHAT ARE YOUR CHOICES?

Finding adequate day care is still a problem. Despite the increase of women in the work force, there are few accommodations for the working mother. As yet we have no governmental programs for child care. Support groups and educational Mom-and-tot classes for mothers and children are held almost exclusively during daytime hours, so a working mother has little opportunity to share experiences with other women.

If a child is sick and both parents work, one parent—usually the mother—must take time off from the job. Day-care centers and nursery schools will not accept that responsibility. One of my dreams for the years to come is day care for children when they have minor acute illnesses. This might be arranged through community hospitals. The center should be staffed by a nurse and several aides, with a pediatrician on call.

I also hope that large corporations will provide more facilities for day care within their organizations. Breast-feeding mothers could then feed their infants without disrupting their work schedules, and mothers would be available if a child became ill or injured.

The ideal solution to child care would be two parents with different work schedules, but we're a long way from that ideal. However, since these are mainly considerations for the future, working parents of young children have to make do with some compromise solutions.

One solution is for mothers to work part-time, perhaps evenings and weekends. Child-care responsibilities are then shared between the two people most concerned. When fathers are totally in charge, they can have the delightful experience of really getting to know their infants. All the fathers in my practice who have child-care responsibilities seem to thrive on the experience.

Another close-to-ideal solution is to have a grandparent or other trusted relative as caretaker. Some of my patients have said that they wouldn't have considered returning to work if their parents hadn't been there to help. But many grandparents are still working themselves and others live in different parts of the country, so this arrangement is rarely possible.

An individual sitter in your own home is another possibility. You may be able to find such a person through a local senior-citizen center or church, through domestic placement agencies, or by placing your own newspaper advertisement. It doesn't matter if the house is kept spotless or even if the caregiver speaks English. In fact, a foreign housekeeper or sitter gives your child the chance to learn a second language. The sitter should know enough English to communicate about issues of daily care and understand what to do in emergencies. But the most important point is that the person be mature and reliable, warm and loving. You may need to interview a number of people before finding the right one.

A neighbor or licensed sitter who provides care for a small number of children in her home can be a good solution. Some of my mothers place ads in the local paper and interview applicants at their homes. We even use my office as a clearing house: prospective sitters and mothers looking for child care post notices on the bulletin board in my waiting room.

It is advisable to interview the prospective sitter at her home with your child present. See how the sitter organizes the day for the other children. Notice if snacks are available, estimate if the group is small enough so that one person can give everybody personal attention, and observe the sitter's behavior toward all the children in her care, including the way she initially relates to your own child. With this kind of observation, you should be reassured that you're making a good choice.

The least desirable, but also the least expensive, option is a large group day-care center.

When you're selecting a day-care center, give close attention to the physical setup of the building: Are older children and infants separated, or are toddlers being clobbered by larger preschoolers? Are there safe areas where diapers can be changed? Are the toys of older children that might be dangerous for infants kept in a separate place? Evaluate the nature of the care with your growing child in mind: Are the day's activities planned in advance and varied according to the age of the children? Are passive infants given as much attention as demanding ones? Is the selection of toys appropriate for each age, and is there enough play space for each child? There should be facilities where meals and snacks can be prepared, and kitchen areas should be neat and clean.

Before and after you enroll your child at any day-care center, visit at unscheduled times—say at 10:00 A.M. or 2:00 P.M.—when parents are not necessarily expected. You should always be welcomed, and there should be absolutely no time when a parent is discouraged from visiting.

Toddlers should have a schedule of activities during the day. Notice whether caregivers are sensitive to babies' individual needs. Children who need a lot of holding and comforting should receive it. The quiet, undemanding child should be actively sought out since that child might easily be overlooked. Babies have their individual cycles of play and rest; when babies are ready to play, someone should be there to play with them.

For children under two, there should be no less than one caregiver for every three children. For children over three, one caregiver for four or five children is adequate.

Once you decide on a sitter or center, accustom your child gradually to the new environment before you return to work. Let the child stay at the center for longer and longer periods of time over a week or two. If you do this in a smooth, gradual way, your child should have no problem accepting the separation of an entire day.

Once your child is enrolled at a center, talk frequently to

the staff members and ask in the morning what is being planned for the day. When you return in the evening, ask what kind of day your child had. This will indicate how tired, stimulated, or cranky your child might be for the rest of the evening, and you'll also have an idea of how good a job the caregivers are doing. Did your son or daughter have a good nap, eat a hearty lunch, or have conflict with other children? The staff should be responsive to parents' requests and concerns, and aware that the working mother needs to feel that she is part of her child's day, even *in absentia.*

Trust your child's reactions. Reluctance to enter a new situation is normal. But if the child repeatedly resists returning to a day-care situation, assume that there's something wrong and consider making other arrangements.

Mark, one of my patients, cried every morning when he was dropped off at day care. At first his mother thought his distress was due to her return to work, but when he was still crying and holding back after several weeks, she consulted me. She was puzzled and worried. The caretaker was certainly qualified, fond of her son, and took excellent care of the other children. The mother had visited this sitter's home at various times and saw a happy, well-organized place.

There seemed nothing wrong, and Mark couldn't tell his mother exactly what was bothering him. Even so, I suggested that she find a new sitter, and she did. Now Mark willingly goes to the new person every morning.

We will never know precisely what happened. Perhaps personal chemistry was at work here. What's important is that Mark communicated his distress to his mother, she listened, and he was allowed to move to a happier situation.

No matter how well-organized the environment, there is one problem when any group of small children is together: the risk of contagion. Day-care centers have always been a cafeteria for viruses and bacteria. Minor viral infections such as colds, flu, vomiting, and diarrhea proliferate wherever children congregate.

More significantly, day-care centers have become breeding grounds for mini-epidemics of infections which were formerly unusual in babies and small children. For example, it was once thought that a parasite called *Giardia lamblia* infected only campers who drank from polluted streams, but now it is a common infestation in day-care centers. No matter how assiduously adult workers wash their hands after contact with individual children, the organism breeds on toys and play surfaces. *Giardia* causes a chronic, annoying diarrhea, and the organism may be difficult to eradicate. Some day-care centers have been temporarily closed because of such epidemics.

Lice, scabies, and several other infections also spread easily in day-care centers. In centers that include children who aren't yet toilet-trained, there may be cases of hepatitis and other intestinally transmitted infections. These can then be transmitted to other family members.

In presenting this picture, I don't mean to say that group day-care centers shouldn't exist, nor are they necessarily unsanitary. No facility serving a number of children can hope to achieve a perfect health standard. You should simply be aware that putting a child into group day care may involve time off from work while a child is recovering from minor illnesses. However, the practicality and the economic saving of group day care may still make the choice acceptable to you.

THE SEPARATION FROM YOUR CHILD

When mothers return to work, they may experience a sense of loss, missing contact with their child and missing some of the joy of motherhood.

Women who are still breast-feeding have a chance to partly assuage some of that loss, for nursing a baby in the evening after work gives both mother and child fifteen or twenty minutes of intimate reunion. It also allows the mother to sit quietly and enjoy one of the most physically pleasurable human experiences. It's understandable that it may be difficult for a mother to leave a small child in the care of another person. But this does not necessarily affect or dilute the mother-child relationship. Child care can, however, create an interesting double bind for a woman if she feels competitive with an outside caregiver. While a mother may want her child to love the caregiver, she may also resent that love. Such feelings are natural, and no harm is done unless the mother pulls away from her child emotionally because of that jealousy. Mother is always Mother to a baby or child, no matter how beloved the other caregiver may be. A child can love others without threatening the love between mother and child.

Some of the studies examining the effects of day care, especially those of a few years ago, were conducted with an initial bias against working mothers. The truth is that there are no good studies showing either benefit or harm over the long term when stable, loving day care is substituted for maternal care. In my opinion, with a *loving* caregiver, a child can only benefit by having more people to love and be loved by, especially in this age of isolated families, far from grandparents, aunts, uncles, and cousins. The mother-child bond is never weakened by a caregiver; children never confuse others with mother. Toddlers in day care easily form multiple attachments without adversely affecting their love for their mothers. There is enough love to go around, and children need as much as you, your family, and your friends can give them.

In fact, an adult who cares for children during the day and knows they will be leaving at five may be more patient with the child, more available to the child, and a better caretaker than the parent who is there twenty-four hours a day.

FOURTEEN

Introducing the Second Child: The Invasion of the Mommy Snatcher

AS THE PARENTS OF a beautiful two year old, you've now learned, through on-the-job training, a great deal about the joys and responsibilities of having a baby. Perhaps, over these two years, you've been discussing whether or not you should have another child. You may already have decided to do so, and your own parents may even be influencing you—they're eager for more grandchildren. Many factors contribute to a couple's decision to have children: factors related to work, money, the time you feel you should have together—in brief, your general life priorities. But the main consideration is: How many children can you care for adequately, in a loving, responsible way?

My husband says that having a first child is like sailing along freely in the sea of life and suddenly having an anchor drop overboard—not an unwelcomed anchor, but an anchor nonetheless. Your life settles into a new routine. After two years, the members of your little family have accommodated to each other, and you're all unbelievably happy. Then the second child comes along. This child doesn't change your lives the way the first one does. The second anchor slows you down a little bit more, but not as drastically as the first.

True though this may be, if your decision is in favor of a single child, I think you'll be encouraged by recent research. Only children are not necessarily spoiled, lonely, overindulged, or at a social disadvantage later in life. In fact, in her book *The Joy of the Only Child,* Ellen Peck cites studies showing that only children may even be better adjusted, with higher self-esteem and better interpersonal relationships, than children with siblings. There are certain advantages to not having to protect toys and territory from usurpation by a brother or sister.

At the same time, siblings do add a great deal to a child's life. If you have brothers or sisters yourself, you know that when you grow up with siblings, you learn the importance of cooperation, loyalty, and tolerance. There are many factors that influence how siblings will feel about each other throughout life—gender and age differences, personality differences, relationships with parents—and with these various contributing factors, it's almost impossible to predict what future relationships will be. We'll concentrate here on the effects of a new baby in the house may have on a first child under the age of four.

Why do I call the second child "the mommy snatcher"? A first child has had undivided attention, and, to a small child, attention is love. When Mommy brings a new baby home from the hospital, the first child has to compete for that attention. That's what makes all the fuss about sibling rivalry. Not only is there new competition, but it's unfair competition—number two is a warm little bundle of joy that everybody falls in love with, so, of course, number one feels somewhat left out or angry. *This is normal behavior!* The best thing you can do for number one is to reassure this child of your love: "Just because Mommy brought home a new baby doesn't mean Mommy loves you less."

Throughout this chapter I'll offer tips on how you can demonstrate that reassurance in words and actions. Take comfort in the fact that the problem diminishes as more children enter the family: a second child has much less trouble with the introduction of a third, because mom's attention was already divided.

THE SPACING OF CHILDREN

Is there an ideal spacing for children in the same family? Children who are close in age may give each other more support and companionship than those who are separated by many years. However, although they may be good playmates and friends, children who are close in age may also be more competitive for parental attention. If the first child is old enough to verbalize feelings and old enough to be reasoned with, a new sibling may be less threatening, but the children's relationship may not be as close. When parents consult me, I tell them that I think three or four years is a good interval between children.

The four year old has a stable, well-established relationship with the parents and has interests outside the home—other playmates or friends at nursery school—but is not so much older than the second child that they can't be good friends while growing up. A child this age can talk about feelings and desires better than a two year old.

I may make recommendations about spacing of children, but they certainly don't hold true for everybody. Elaine, herself a mother of four, tells me that when her sister was born nine years later, she felt that her parents were having this baby just for her. The sisters still have an extremely close relationship. Jill, on the other hand, says that she and her two sisters, all one year apart, have grown up with remarkable closeness.

My co-author Kathy has brothers who are very close in age: twenty minutes apart. She's eighteen months older than her twin brothers, and they've always gotten along very well. In fact, Kathy was the only one—except for their parents—who could tell which twin was which. At school the twins wore shirts with their names sewed on for identification and once as a joke traded shirts. Kathy recalls feeling very important when she could correct the confused kindergarten teacher by saying: "No, that's Tommy and that's Bobby." She also feels that her mother did an excellent job of praising each child for his or her special qualities and providing an environment where those qualities could flourish. All three children grew up to be intelligent, highly motivated adults.

The fact is, there's no way to know what sort of a relationship will develop between siblings. My advice is to establish your priorities with your partner. Can you afford a second child now, or will you be able to handle it better in two or three years? If you work, will that be a good time for you to take time off? Is your age and the biological clock a factor?

PREPARING THE FIRST CHILD FOR THE NEW BABY

There are several things you can do to prepare your first child for the arrival of a new baby. Although the full impact won't be felt until the baby actually arrives, making the first child feel involved and special will help ensure a positive experience.

First of all, announce the coming birth as early as possible so the child can have several months to anticipate it and become accustomed to the idea. Two-year-old Rebecca repeatedly tells me that her sister is in Mommy's tummy. She doesn't actually know that it will be a girl, although she and her mother's obstetrician have a running discussion at each visit about the gender of the fetus. More important, however, although Rebecca has no idea what the arrival of a sister will mean to her, she understands that this baby will be welcomed and is eager for the baby. Rebecca's mother has done a good job of preparing her first child for a brother or a sister who will be a companion for Rebecca, not a threat.

Many small children think that the baby in Mommy's tummy is a miniature of themselves and that as soon as the baby is born they will have a playmate. Imagine their disappointment when they see that the new baby isn't even as much fun as a Cabbage Patch doll. Before the birth of the second child, you might plan to visit families with a small baby and use the time to talk about the ways babies are different from big boys and girls. Show the older child what a baby can and cannot do. And remind your child that as soon as the baby grows older, this brother or sister will be a splendid playmate.

Before the birth, you can show a child of three years or more the right way to handle a baby. Buy a special doll that will be the older child's baby, and show the child how to bathe, burp, feed, and change the doll. This not only teaches the child what behaviors will be helpful, it also allows the child to become adept at various activities. The older child can then play alongside Mommy and take care of the doll as Mother cares for the baby, making the child feel more involved and competent. This works best if you introduce the doll long before the birth; once the baby arrives, a doll is a poor substitute for the real thing.

Buy a supply of small gifts to give the older child when friends bring presents to your home for the new arrival. If the visitors are not thoughtful enough to remember the older child, you can avoid jealousy by having a gift handy. This could be a present "from the new baby to big sister" or a special surprise from Mommy to number one.

If you want to use the first child's crib for the baby, you can avoid making number one feel displaced by changing beds before the second one arrives. Take the child shopping for a new bed, and let the child test them all and participate in the final choice.

On another shopping trip, allow number one to choose clothes and toys for the new baby, and make a point of letting the child select the outfit in which you'll bring the baby home.

Include your first child in packing the suitcase you will take to the hospital and in setting up the room for the new baby. Your older child may be able to help put diapers away and arrange clothing, some of which will inevitably be some of the child's own former outfits.

A mother I know prepared a tape of her voice singing her child's favorite songs, which her daughter could play on her indestructible Fisher-Price tape player if she became lonely for Mommy while Mommy was in the hospital.

Nearly all hospitals allow siblings to visit, although the hours may be limited. The hospital where I work not only offers a tour for prospective parents, but a "tyke hike." Older children are taken on a tour of the nursery and postpartum area so they'll feel familiar with the wards when they visit the mother.

The first child will necessarily be deprived of mother's company during labor, delivery, and the postpartum period. I encourage mothers to leave the hospital as soon as possible, whether or not there are children at home; the home atmosphere is always more comfortable, and the right environment for rest and nursing are better achieved in familiar surroundings. With a first child at home, it's even more important to return as quickly as is medically sensible.

No matter how long or short the hospital stay, keep the first child at home rather than in the home of friends or relatives. If the father has already been a prominent part of the child's life, the time alone with Daddy will be a special treat, and offsetting the temporary loss of Mommy. Encourage the child to visit the hospital and to telephone whenever he or she wants to call. Mother should also call home spontaneously and frequently.

A few years ago, as I was making rounds in the early evening, I entered a room in which two of my mothers were recuperating. On the first bed sat the father with his arm around his wife, while uncle and grandmother sat beside the bed. On the other bed, the mother's two-and-a-half-year-old son played quietly while she stroked his head. I was touched and thought, "This is the way it should be: people you love around you in a relaxed, comfortable atmosphere."

In most hospitals, children can only view the new baby through the nursery window and visit mother only when the baby is not present. This routine is changing slowly, but hospital infection-control committees must first be convinced that relaxing the rules won't increase infection in the nursery. Until this procedure changes, the older child's first direct contact with the new baby is at the time of discharge.

Include number one in the trip home from the hospital so that the child senses that the three of you are adding another member to the family, rather than bringing home an invader.

THE OLDER CHILD AND THE NEWBORN

At first, a new baby is such a novelty and so strange to the older child that there is little difficulty with resentment. More often than not, parents have to keep the curious older child away from the baby. The most common expression on the face of the older child is likely to be wonder, sometimes elation, and occasionally confusion. It's only after number one realizes that feeding the baby not only takes a long time but happens so often that behavior starts to change.

First children are aware that adults praise them for loving behavior toward the baby and may go to great (sometimes theatrical) lengths to demonstrate affection. This first loving behavior is almost always in imitation of adult behavior. "Real" affection develops later.

If the first child has negative feelings, they almost always come out in ways that are not directly related to the baby: the first child may fall down and cry in pain just as the baby is being fed or may break a glass in the kitchen as you prepare to bathe the baby. Show that you do not approve of deliberate misbehavior, and discipline the older child as you always do, but also realize that the unwanted behavior means that the child is asking for additional, personal attention.

Find extra time for the older child—a special story at bedtime or extra time together when the baby sleeps. Leave the baby with Dad while Mom and number one do errands, or hire a sitter for an afternoon regularly and devote that time to your older child.

It also helps to reassure the first child that angry or resentful feelings toward the baby are normal, that sometimes the first child may wish the infant would go back to where it came from. Big sister doesn't always have to feel the way the adults around her feel. It's also important to make clear to a three or four year old that words are not magical, and that saying how you feel won't hurt the baby. The older child can then feel safe enough to say that the baby should be fed to the alligators without being fearful of the consequences. Once these feelings are stated, you can explore them further and reassure number one of your love.

Jeannie, one of the nurses in my office, wishes she had taken four-year-old Michelle's efforts to help with Baby Stacy more seriously. Jeannie regrets now that she didn't allow her firstborn to be more involved when Michelle asked to help with the new baby, for Jeannie thinks it would have given Michelle a more positive experience in the second child's first weeks. Don't force the child to be an aide, but teach the child who wants to learn how to help and accept that help as a great gift. Reinforce it with praise.

Show the older child how to attract the baby's attention, how to tell which toys the baby likes best, how to make faces for the infant to imitate. But remember that no matter how positive and loving the first child may seem toward the newborn, there may be some ambivalence. The first child may be angry with Mom and Dad for introducing number two. Mommy is essential to life and the baby is helpless, so the jealously is directed toward the baby. Never leave the first child alone with the new baby, for that ambivalence may materialize as a mysterious bump on the newborn's head or worse. The mother of three-year-old Matthew found him striking the new baby on the head with a plastic hammer. Thereafter, whenever she had to leave the room, she took the baby along. Traipsing after his mother and brother, Matthew sighed, "I won't hurt the baby." He knew that he did wrong, but his mother was wisely being cautious.

In a few short months a wonderful phenomenon will occur. Over and over parents tell me that there is no one who can make the baby as happy as an older brother or sister. I don't know how babies know that children are more like them than their parents, but they seem to understand right from the start. They have a special response to the older child. A two month old will smile sweetly for Mother or Father, but beam ecstatically, squeal, kick, and giggle for a three-year-old brother or sister.

If you take care to prepare for the new arrival and provide every possible opportunity for involvement in infant care, it will be a rich and rewarding experience for everyone in the family.

Afterword

AS I WAS FINISHING THIS BOOK, I had a particularly delightful conversation with a highly verbal four year old. As we ended our conversation, I said, "You're very special, you know."

Her wise reply was "Everyone's special."

In this book I've talked about the choices you'll have as a parent and some of the options available to you. But, remember, this is a one-way conversation. It's not possible for me to know your situation. You and your child are distinct individuals and a unique combination. Except for material dealing with physical safety and some fundamental health issues such as immunization and the use of medications, there is nothing in this book that should be considered absolute. The most important question to ask yourself is this: Is what you are doing comfortable for you *and* your child? If it is, then you're making the right choice.

I hope I've convinced you that you are the best-equipped person to make decisions about your own baby. There will be times when you may be anxious or confused. You will turn to your own pediatrician for medical counsel, as my patients do with me, and we, as your doctors, will share the joyful times with you.

L.S.

Acknowledgments

SPECIAL THANKS go to our agents, Wendy Weil, Kathy Robbins, and Loretta Fidel, for their enthusiasm and support for the concept of this book; and to our editor, Carol Houck Smith, for her guidance and patience during the writing process. Thanks also to Dianne Woo for research help and to Linda Kamberg de Martinez for manuscript typing.

THIS BOOK would not have been possible without the cooperation of my partner, Albert J. Melaragno, M.D., my colleague Rochelle Feldman, M.D., and the special contribution of Eileen Yager, M.D., and the outstanding women in my office. I am also grateful to Catherine Clark, Ph.D.; the Ritters, the Hills, the Dombeys, the Thornburghs, and countless other patients who have given me the best education a pediatrician ever had.

My husband, Jack Nides, made my hours at the typewriter almost easy; Tina Nides made the book happen. I also want to express my thanks to the producers of "Hour Magazine" —Larry Ferber, Steve Clements, and Marty Berman—as well as to Michael Jackson of ABC Radio, for introducing me to the fun of talking to more than one parent at a time.

L.S.

THE ENCOURAGEMENT of Lourdes Blanco of Caracas, Dr. Jane Rabb at Harvard, and Mr. and Mrs. G. D'Andelot Belin of Cambridge, Massachusetts, has been deeply important to me. These people believed in my goal of a writing career from the start. Miss Gillard at King's Hall in Canada taught me to have the guts to pursue it.

K.M.

Suggested Reading

CHILDBIRTH

Hotchner, Tracy. *Pregnancy and Childbirth.* New York: Avon, 1979. Some sections of this book are out of date, but it is still the most complete source of information about all aspects of childbirth.

Leboyer, Frederick. *Birth without Violence.* New York: Knopf, 1980. A sensitive, enlightening, and easy-to-read book about labor and delivery, focusing on the child's experience.

BREAST FEEDING

La Leche League. *The Womanly Art of Breastfeeding.* Franklin Park, Ill.: 1981. An informative guide to all aspects of breast feeding.

Price, Ann, and Nancy Bamford. *The Breastfeeding Guide for the*

Working Woman. New York: Simon and Schuster, 1983. Practical help for the career woman who wants to breast-feed.

Pryor, Karen. *Nursing Your Baby.* New York: Simon and Schuster, 1973. This one is more supportive of the working woman than the La Leche League book, but not as comprehensive as a reference.

FEEDING SOLIDS

Brody, Jane. *Jane Brody's Nutrition Book.* New York: W. W. Norton, 1981. A comprehensive and sensible guide to family nutrition.

Lansky, Vicky. *Feed Me, I'm Yours.* Deephaven, Minn.: Meadowbrook Press, 1974. Written by a mother and her health-conscious friends who felt there was a need for a book about feeding small children. Contains useful recipes to vary feeding routines.

DEVELOPMENT

Brazelton, T. Berry, M.D. *Infants and Mothers, Individual Differences in Development.* New York: Delacorte Press, 1983. Deals with the wide variations of development based on children's individual characteristics.

Caplan, Frank, ed. *The First Twelve Months of Life.* New York: Perigee Books, 1973.

Caplan, Frank, and Theresa Caplan. *The Second Twelve Months of Life.* New York: Perigee Books, 1977. These two books, written by members of the Princeton Center for Infancy and Early Childhood, are complete and thoughtful discussions of each month of the first two years.

Fraiberg, Selma. *The Magic Years.* New York: Scribners, 1959. This book is dated in some of the material on the newborn, but is important as a sensitive and enjoyable description of what it's like to be a small child.

SIBLINGS

Szasz, Susan, and Elizabeth Talporos. *Sisters, Brothers, and Others.* New York: W. W. Norton, 1984. A beautiful collection of intimate photographs and sensitive text about the many ways families and siblings adapt to a new baby.

Index